Sex Ed, Segregated

Gender and Race in American History

Alison M. Parker, The College at Brockport,
State University of New York
Carol Faulkner, Syracuse University

Sex Ed, Segregated

The Quest for Sexual Knowledge in Progressive-Era America

Courtney Q. Shah

UNIVERSITY OF ROCHESTER PRESS

First published 2015

University of Rochester Press
668 Mt. Hope Avenue, Rochester, NY14620, USA
www.urpress.com
and Boydell & Brewer Limited
PO Box 9, Woodbridge, Suffolk IP12 3DF, UK
www.boydellandbrewer.com

ISBN-13: 978-1-58046-535-9
ISSN: 2152-6400

Library of Congress Cataloging-in-Publication Data

Shah, Courtney Q., author.
   Sex ed, segregated : the quest for sexual knowledge in progressive-era America / Courtney Q. Shah.
      p. ; cm. — (Gender and race in American history, ISSN 2152-6400 ; v. 6)
   Includes bibliographical references and index.
   ISBN 978-1-58046-535-9 (hardcover : alk. paper)
   I. Title. II. Series: Gender and race in American history. 2152-6400
   [DNLM: 1. Sex Education—history—United States. 2. History, 19th Century—United States. 3. History, 20th Century—United States. 4. Racism—history—United States. 5. Sexuality—history—United States. 6. Sexually Transmitted Diseases—prevention & control—United States. HQ 56]
   HQ56
   613.9'6—dc23
                                                            2015012235

A catalogue record for this title is available from the British Library.

This publication is printed on acid-free paper.
Printed and bound by CPI Group (UK) Ltd, Croydon, CR0 4YY.

Contents

Acknowledgments

I could not have completed this book without the support and assistance of many people. My first and principal debt is to Dr. Landon R. Y. Storrs, who advised me throughout my graduate career and beyond. Thank you to the University of Rochester Press, particularly Sonia Kane, Alison M. Parker, and Carol Faulkner, as well as my anonymous readers, who provided invaluable critiques of my manuscript and pushed me to think more deeply and produce a stronger work.

Many colleagues near and far shaped my thinking through coursework, conversation, and collegiality. Roberta Bivins, Kathleen Brosnan, Sarah Fishman, Karl Ittmann, Jacqueline Jones, Jane Kamensky, Craig Livingston, Steven Mintz, Martin Pernick, Joseph Pratt, Helen K. Valier, Eric Walther, and Michael Willrich each contributed in their own ways. I am grateful for the inestimable gift of my writing sisterhood! Marjorie Denise Brown, LaGuana Gray, Theresa Jach, and Angela Murphy provided emotional as well as intellectual support. They contributed suggestions on manuscripts, supportive emails, and lunches out so that none of us would become isolated and buried in our work. Emily Straus told me I could (and should) publish the book and continues to take good care of me from afar. In addition, Sonia Hernandez, Clayton Lust, and Albert Rodriguez provided a sounding board at critical moments in the process. My colleagues in the Department of Social Sciences at Lower Columbia College, especially Dennis Shaw, provided valuable support. Kristy Thompson and Neel Mehta read parts of the manuscript and provided me access to the American Film Institute silent film database. Maulin Shah enabled my work throughout the process.

The Department of History at the University of Houston assisted me through its generous financial support in the form of a King Fellowship and a Murry Miller travel grant to complete my research. I would like to thank the University of Minnesota for the Clarke Chambers Fellowship and David Klaassen and his staff at the Social Welfare History Archives for their expert assistance during my research trip. Lower Columbia College provided a travel grant, enabling me to present at the Organization of American Historians conference, which reinvigorated the project. I would also like to thank the Houston Academy of Medicine library, Bexar County Clerk Gerry Rickhoff and his staff at the Bexar County Courthouse, and the staff at the Institute of Texan

Cultures at the University of Texas at San Antonio. The wonderful people at the University of Houston interlibrary loan department allowed me to access a wide range of materials from across the nation. I would like to thank the staff of Portland State University Millar Library and the Lower Columbia College Library for their assistance. And I thank the University of Texas Press for their permission to reproduce in chapter 6 portions of my article "'Against Their Own Weakness': Policing Sexuality and Women in San Antonio, Texas, during World War I," *Journal of the History of Sexuality* 19, no. 3 (2010): 458–82. © 2010 by the University of Texas Press.

More personally, I want to express my gratitude to Camie Wilson, who takes wonderful care of my children (and me). Thank you to my parents, Jim and Maureen Forsloff, for supporting my education in every way. And last, to Maya and Kamran: Mama wrote a book!

Introduction

In 1903, concerned newlyweds or curious adolescents may have found themselves furtively reading advice manuals on courtship, marriage, and sex. A proper young African American lady may have received *Golden Thoughts on Chastity and Procreation*, written by a married couple in conjunction with a medical doctor, to learn the most healthful and responsible way to live her life. The book aimed to teach Victorian, middle-class sexual respectability. It included paradoxical messages on sexuality and procreation: "Prudery says: Keep still; do not talk about our sexual natures. Duty says: Cry aloud; let the truth be known; publish it to the world; save the people from pollution and destruction; from death. God says: 'My people are destroyed for lack of knowledge.'—Hosea iv. 6."[1] The book provided explicit discussion of puberty, sexual intercourse, reproduction, and venereal diseases (VD). It combined the science of the time with a solid moral and Christian justification. Sexual knowledge, it argued, was a blessing to both good health and morality.

But the story of *Golden Thoughts* was more complicated. On the other side of town, outside of the Jim Crow neighborhoods, white audiences could furtively read the same book, this time entitled *Social Purity, or, the Life of the Home and Nation*.[2] The publishers did not edit the content of the book, changing only the title, the introduction (*Golden Thoughts* opened with an introduction by a noted black physician, Henry Rutherford Butler), and the illustrations.[3] Drawings of black families in one and white families in the other made clear who the intended audience was. It appeared that blacks and whites had much in common and faced many of the same difficulties, but book publishers and sex educators were determined to keep them separate. Why?

The titles themselves suggest racial assumptions. *Golden Thoughts* is far more euphemistic, stressing "chastity" and "procreation" as the main tenets of sexual education. The stress on chastity implies the politics of respectability, so crucial to black middle class status, and defines sexuality as procreative rather than pleasurable. *Social Purity* links this individual book to the emerging national "social purity" movement and indeed suggests the importance of the nation in its title. Readers of *Social Purity* could improve the life of the home and the nation, institutions to reproduce (white) American culture.[4]

The separate publication of these two books demonstrates several points. It shows the depth of racial segregation in the United States at the turn of the twentieth century. It illustrates the aspirations of the black middle class. Yet it also suggests the desire for, and existence of, a single moral standard for whites and blacks, at least in prescriptive literature. Whites may have believed that their moral and sexual behavior separated them from blacks, but, in fact, the middle classes of both races consumed the same advice and aspired to act in the same ways.[5] Finally, it shows that sex education and sexual knowledge played a role in establishing respectable morality.

Both books utilized typical Progressive reform strategies. *Golden Thoughts* and *Social Purity* advocated education and publicity as the solution to social problems. Both recognized the importance of science while at the same time appealing to the Bible as the highest authority—the title *Golden Thoughts* could also connote the importance of the Golden Rule. Both combined pessimism about contemporary society with optimism that through a few key reforms, the world could be remade and salvation could be attained. And both saw education—the power of knowledge—as vital to that salvation.

Sex education has the potential to empower people with knowledge to make good decisions about their bodies and their relationships. It can increase health and wellness and free people from pernicious, uninformed stereotypes. In the early twentieth century, it occasionally did these things. But, more commonly, Progressive sex education information bolstered existing stereotypes. It normalized white male (middle class) sexuality and pathologized any departures from the white male norm.[6] It was rife with eugenic language about improving the race—usually with obvious connotations of racial superiority. And it was used to justify existing political hierarchies in the name of science and morality. Both medical expertise and moral authority backed specious claims about who was and was not able to learn about sex. However, those shunted to the side of white middle-class male authority fought back, challenging and altering the discourse to improve their own conditions. The sex education movement thus provides a window through which scholars can view the conflict between reformers and conservatives, whites and nonwhites, men and women, and the way these conflicts affected power relationships between different groups.

The sex education movement, growing by leaps and bounds at the beginning of the twentieth century, emerged out of the reform atmosphere of the Progressive Era. Sex education advocates wanted to use science and knowledge to improve society. Through expert leadership, publication, and ubiquitous education, social hygienists believed they could solve the problem of marital incompatibility, eliminate venereal diseases, end prostitution, and save the next generation's bodies and souls. Such grandiose goals depended on a positive view of people's rational nature. But social hygienists and other Progressives did not see all people as being equally rational or equally salvageable. They believed that middle-class whites had a greater capacity than others to practice sexual morality. As such, the sex education movement often overlapped with the eugenics movement, which sought to improve "the race" by encouraging the right people to breed and discouraging the unfit. Eugenicists used slippery definitions of race, though, which could be limited to only white or only Anglo-Saxon citizens.

Hierarchies based on white supremacy and patriarchy played a central role in the formation of the sex education movement in the United States in the early twentieth century. Social and medical assumptions about the audience's race, gender, and class identity affected both the material that reformers considered appropriate to teach and the pedagogical method they used. The national social hygiene movement tended to target white middle-class men and, to a lesser extent, the white working class, drawing on both social and medical beliefs about physiology and disease trajectory to justify its disinterest in racial minorities. *Social Purity* could be viewed as the mainstream curriculum—*Golden Thoughts* a way to make a larger profit by repackaging the same material to expand its audience. Yet the two separate titles reinforced the illusion that the curriculum differed according to race. The biology may not have been different between white and black, but the social context was. Even more than race, reformers' assumptions about male and female sexuality differed substantially based on nineteenth-century assumptions about sexual development, which influenced the sorts of instructional methods advocated for girls and boys.

Likewise, assumptions about identity shaped conservative resistance to sex education, both in and out of schools. The conflict over sex education represented a broader response, both positive and negative, to the changing role schools, institutions, and the government played in family life during the Progressive Era. Many would have simply preferred to avoid the topic altogether, linking ignorance with innocence in all matters sexual.

By the beginning of World War I, the US military had to face the reality of surprisingly high rates of venereal disease among recruits. This challenged the prevailing conspiracy of silence on all things sexual. Framing sex education as a matter of national security, the federal government adopted a more active role in presenting sex education to soldiers and civilians. The identity of the audience continued to dominate the discourse on the appropriateness of the material and the content of the material itself. While the military hoped to diminish the class differences among soldiers, it maintained clear boundaries based on race and gender. The study of sex education shows how the advent of "modern" social sensibilities, especially regarding sex, failed to challenge existing social hierarchies.

Human sexuality is not ahistorical—although biology or anatomy may not have changed drastically, cultural understandings of sex, and assumptions about appropriate sexual behavior and how it is learned, have. Scholarship in the past several decades has shown that historical circumstances shaped sexual beliefs, behaviors, and attitudes, making the history of sexuality an established field of scholarship.[7] The scholarship on sex education has broadened our understanding of the ways in which evolving scientific information (including popular pseudoscience like eugenics) and societal pressures affected the most intimate aspects of people's lives.[8]

To see the roots of American sex education, we must look outside of the schoolroom. The few early efforts to implement sex education in the schools classes met fierce resistance. Instead, reformers turned to extracurricular programs such as the Boy Scouts of America (BSA), the Young Men's Christian Association (YMCA), and the popular club movement of the Progressive Era. Public debate over previously "private sphere" issues characterized the Progressive Era. Everything from clean milk campaigns to the establishment of settlement houses demonstrated the shifting of "private" concerns to public (if not governmental) activism. Immigration restriction and eugenic legislation were two examples of the state intruding on who could qualify as an American.[9]

World War I catalyzed a rapid change of course. Patriotism and military readiness played a critical role in establishing the necessity of an active sex education campaign. Under the auspices of national emergency, the federal government stepped in to cope with social problems like venereal disease. As such, federal sexual education policies accorded with an expansion of a more active (and intrusive) government over the course of the twentieth century.[10]

Changing times increased the demand for sex education, but they also changed the way sex education was delivered. Increasing literacy rates prompted an expanding publishing business.[11] Immigration prompted a demand for material in languages other than English. Cheap newspaper and magazine printing technologies allowed for widespread distribution of shorter articles. Apart from the written word, early sex education efforts employed the "gee whiz" factor of new media like motion pictures. Visual popular culture reflected a pleasure-based sexual discourse in the Progressive Era in entertainment, one that could be turned to educational purposes. The entertainment and novelty of new media also helped to reach nonliterate audiences.[12] The inclusion of sex education films reveals the public's uncertainty about the propriety and usefulness of new visual media, especially among multiracial or mixed-sex audiences. Visual presentations could contribute to learning, but they could also be "racy" in a way that written words were not.

Reacting to the current debate over sex education, scholars have reemphasized the connections between school-based sex education and sexual culture. School-based sex educators attempted to quash adolescent sexuality, seeing it as something far different and more threatening than adult sexuality. However, school curricula had little success in "curing," or at least making invisible, adolescent sexuality through education. Throughout the twentieth century, parents, schools, students, and the federal government have battled over the content and messaging of sex education curriculum. There was no linear progression from reticence to full disclosure; rather, there was (and continues to be) a strong conflict among interest groups over sex education.

My research demonstrates how American racism complicated sex educa-tion. African Americans resisted racist sexual stereotypes by providing alter-native medical and social theories, attempting to redefine sexual knowledge within their own communities. By establishing their expertise as scientific and moral authorities, black sex educators challenged so-called biological dif-ferences between the races and uplifted the race by supporting middle-class respectability. Segregation was ultimately a strong force in Progressive reform, including sex education.

Segregation could divide audiences along racial or gender lines, which occasionally resulted in empowering knowledge. Sex education sometimes provided unexpected freedoms for women.[13] Female advocates of explicit sex education pushed for forthright sexual information in order to destroy the appeal of commercialized prostitution and pornography.[14] Conversely, women of the 1920s claimed sexual knowledge, rather than reticence, dissemblance, or "passionlessness," to demand greater social and political equality or to capi-talize on the sexual marketplace.[15] My study shifts this concept back into the Progressive Era, arguing that sex education for girls had the potential for radi-cal feminist results despite the conservative demands that sex education be limited to marital propriety.

But uniting all women in a feminist crusade for educational opportunity was only a pipe dream. Class and racial lines still divided women, preventing the establishment of a common cause. Women purity activists and medical doctors vied for power over sex education, often at odds with each other's aims. The sexual double standard, which many purity activists wished to see disappear as men were held to the same standard as women, instead shifted to allowing women greater sexual leeway. But the double standard survived (mostly) intact. Especially in the context of the predominantly male world of military and political programs, the pragmatism of a medical program that protected male sexual prerogative divided the social hygiene movement along gender and generational lines. Women's racial and class identities divided their loyalties rather than uniting their efforts at establishing women's equal participation in medical and social reform organizations. What is more, the "old-fashioned" purity advocates who sought to reach female audiences after World War I were viewed as quaint and ineffective.[16]

Building upon a rich scholarship on sexuality, education, and identity, *Sex Ed, Segregated* argues that the quest for sexual knowledge in the United States took different forms based on the intended audience. Reformers and instruc-tors taught middle-class youth, African Americans, and World War I soldiers different stories, for different reasons. Reformers' assumptions about their audience's place in the political hierarchy played a crucial role in the develop-ment of a mainstream sex education movement by the 1920s. Therefore, what could have been a revolutionary way of empowering people was more often used to reinforce power relations. Reformers used sex education to establish social control, segregation, and their own expertise during the Progressive Era. The debate between biological and cultural differences permeated both the social and medical debates over sexuality. For instance, using the documents of the National Medical Association (NMA), the preeminent organization for black health professionals, my work highlights how alternative institutions opposed scientific racism and how the categories of class and gender worked in conjunction with or in opposition to categories of race. Examination of "character-building" organizations like the YMCA and the BSA shows how the white middle-class ideal reflected cultural assumptions about sexuality and formed an aspirational model for upward mobility to those not in the privileged group, such as immigrant or working class youth. In addition, the battle over policing young women's sexual behavior during World War I pitted middle-class women against their working-class counterparts. Identity shaped beliefs about sexual behavior, education, and even physiology. The intersection of race, gender, and class formed the backbone of Progressive-Era debates over sex education, the policing of sexuality, and the prevention of venereal disease.

I have set forth this argument in seven chapters. Chapter 1 examines the foundation of the American Social Hygiene Association (ASHA), which united the religiously inspired purity movement and the medical community's concern over venereal disease. Despite its efforts at building a nationwide organization, ASHA and its predecessors attracted only a limited audience. White, middle-class, native-born, and mostly from the Northeast, the social hygiene movement lacked sustained development in the South and in many rural areas, due in large part to the organization's racial and eugenic assumptions.

Chapter 2 discusses the struggles over placing sex education in front of an audience prior to World War I. After initial attempts in Chicago in 1913 met with failure, ASHA backpedaled from school inclusion. Even if sex education had found a welcome home in the schools, it would have been limited on the basis of race, region, and class. Reformers who had previously debated sexual purity versus sexual hygiene shifted to battle whether the curriculum should be in schools or homes.

As school-based curricula met with obstacles, alternate institutions took up the mantle of sex education, further shaping the curriculum. Chapter 3 examines how character-building organizations like the Boy Scouts and the YMCA defined adolescence and character, thereby limiting sex education to a predominantly white male audience. Many reformers shied away from demanding education for girls beyond the basics of hygiene, assuming that knowledge would be unnecessary for girls, who supposedly lacked sexual desire. Conflict between ideals and reality created concerns over girls' sexual and class identities.

If sex education became popular among white character-building organizations, the debate within medical circles kept the matter of race in the vanguard. Chapter 4 analyzes the discourse of race and venereal diseases. White doctors, often claiming expertise based on their identity as southerners, built on a history of colonial medicine that relegated blacks to the realm of untreatable, hopeless cases. Therefore, many argued that sex education for African Americans was a waste of resources. The expanding black medical profession and middle class repudiated sexual stereotyping based on race. In response to a white medical discourse that attacked black sexual morality, black professionals often embraced sexual Victorianism and redefined sexual behavior as a function of class and gender, using sex education as a way to uplift the race into middle-class respectability, while at the same time criticizing the lower classes for dangerous sexual behaviors.

While not erasing the debates over class and race, World War I provided a turning point in public opinion about the necessity of sex education. Chapter 5 examines the American Plan, the government's effort to provide education, medical treatment, law enforcement, and recreation to encourage sexual purity and halt the spread of venereal disease. The program contained inconsistencies in its implementation based on both race and class. Because of segregation and biological assumptions about of black male sexuality, the military provided blacks with less rigorous educational programs, fewer recreational options, and less medical treatment. Lectures, pamphlets, and visual media linked patriotism and sexual purity to white middle-class male identity, further differentiating among racial and class groups and leaving women out.

Chapter 6 extends the analysis of wartime sex education programs to the civilian population, particularly women. Focusing on vice enforcement around army bases, the chapter argues that the wartime emergency provided national and municipal authorities with the rationale to detain and punish women, especially working-class women and women of color, for suspected sexual impropriety. I recount the battle between Progressive women's desire for female protection and their desire for autonomy. Reformers in cities like San Antonio, Texas, used class- and race-based language and punishment to police sexuality in their town. This included the establishment of police matrons, female police officers, women's educational programs, and detention homes for female sexual delinquents. Assumptions about women's sexual nature divided women rather than uniting them.

The end of the war marked a major change in American cultural life. Chapter 7 examines the expansion of education for teens and young adults in high schools and colleges during the "roaring twenties." Yet the marital adjustment classes of the 1920s expressed conservatives' desire to contain and domesticate the ever-expanding sexual culture of the 1920s. Young people, responding to greater leisure time, disposable income, freedom through automobiles, and peer group socialization, embraced the sexual revolution of the 1910s. The flapper came of age, attending necking parties with a flask hidden under her skirt. Her high school or college classroom taught her one set of lessons, while movies, magazines, celebrity culture, and her peer group taught her another.

The legacy of the Progressive-Era sex education movement should be understood as reform rather than revolution. Sex education reform provided useful, empowering knowledge to some, but it contained a darker message as well. *Sex Ed, Segregated* demonstrates that the sex education movement divided audiences into the salvageable and the hopeless. Sex education had the potential (and occasionally the glimmers of reality) to empower people. But hierarchies of race, class, and gender remained rigid in both access to knowledge and public and private power relations. The "progressive" reform efforts imposed middle-class morality, encouraged segregation, and coerced behavior through scientific prescription.

Between the 1890s and the 1920s, greater public acceptance of sexual discourse paved the way for broader sex education programs. But reformers still limited the curriculum to "normal" adjustment and heterosexual marriage. Identity markers such as race, class, and gender continued to play a significant role in determining what a person learned, why, and how. This legacy continues even into the twenty-first century, as the United States continues to cling to hierarchies based on our (outdated and unscientific) assumptions about sex.

Chapter One

The Origins of the Sex Education Movement

Denslow Lewis, a Chicago physician, presented a controversial paper at an 1899 meeting of the American Medical Association (AMA). His work focused on how sex education could improve marital satisfaction, especially for women who suffered physical discomfort during sexual intercourse. The response from his colleagues was less than positive. Most present echoed the sentiments of gynecologist Howard Kelly, who commented, "[The topic's] discussion is attended with filth and we besmirch ourselves by discussing it in public." The AMA allowed the paper's inclusion in the annual session but later refused to publish the paper in their journal, noting the controversial nature of Lewis's work.[1]

The twentieth century dawned with even physicians hesitant to discuss sex education. Yet Progressive reformers prided themselves on exposing and solving the nation's problems. Could they do it with what social purity activists believed was the biggest problem of all, sex? According to Delcevare King, a wealthy philanthropist and social purity activist, the best way to improve America was to start a nationwide campaign to change sexual behavior. In 1910, he wrote to New York dermatologist Dr. Prince A. Morrow. Morrow had been working for more than a decade to both bring European venereology work to the United States and to advocate for better sexual hygiene education. Morrow attended international conferences on venereal diseases and was eager to share his knowledge with the American public. King wrote, "That idea of a National Organization as the centre of a National Movement for Sex Education gripped hold of me last night and so I am having to write you this letter." He suggested the need to end the "conspiracy of silence," which he called the "most terrible failure of our civilization." He wanted Morrow to piece together the organization and looked to no less a figure than former president Theodore Roosevelt to be the group's executive. King offered his own money to begin the endowment, saying, "I know something of the difficulties of money raising but I also know what can be done where there is a concrete plan and where earnest men who believe in it, will give most of their time for a brief period toward putting it through."[2]

Morrow wrote back immediately: "My own idea has been that this movement would be of slow growth, evolutionary rather than revolutionary, but I am fully persuaded that your idea of doing something big is the correct one."[3] Morrow's response highlights the difficulties he perceived in convincing the nation to accept what King wanted. Was the United States ready for sex education? Morrow had written the previous year to another eager contributor, "When the public is more fully educated, the ideals you have in view may be realized."[4] He hoped to create a movement akin to that of Jean-Alfred Fournier, the French physician who had published both academic texts and educational pamphlets on syphilis for young people. Morrow thought that if sex education advocates pushed too hard, conservative Americans would reject them outright. A Progressive who believed in reform rather than revolution, Morrow had himself experienced difficulty when trying to broach the subject of sex in the medical profession. He helped shape the American Social Hygiene Association (ASHA) as a group that wished to present sex education to American society in a way that did not threaten the nation's sensibilities.[5] Through the formation of ASHA, purity reformers and physicians worked together to find a way to present a palatable form of sex education to Americans. Despite multifarious strategies and theories, the sex education movement remained extremely limited in its scope before World War I.

Sexual Discourse at the Turn of the Century

The leaders of the sex education movement found it daunting at the turn of the twentieth century to challenge "Victorianism," the catchall term for nineteenth-century Anglo-American attitudes embraced by the growing urban middle class. Foremost among these attitudes, the middle class embraced respectability, defined by sexual continence, privacy in home life, and the repression of public discussion of sex or reproduction. Dr. Maurice Bigelow, a professor of biology and director of Columbia University's Teachers College, wrote in 1914, "The time-honored policy has been one of silence and mystery concerning all things sexual."[6] In fact, "Victorian" America was not nearly as reticent about sexual discourse as cultural stereotypes or Sigmund Freud would have us believe. A culture of self-proclaimed bohemians celebrated sexual emancipation from cultural norms in the late nineteenth century. Radical feminist Victoria Woodhull, for instance, challenged sexual standards both through her own life and by exposing sexual misconduct among others.[7] Bigelow and other commentators may have exaggerated the silence on sexual topics in order to demonstrate their own propriety or candor. It was not silence but an emerging medicalization of sexuality that marked the nineteenth century, as sex became a topic of fierce medical and sociological debate. Discussion of sexuality, both normal and abnormal, was rampant in the popular culture. But legal censorship and social ostracism worked against the medical necessity or commercial appeal of sex education books.[8] Many authors hoped to limit distribution to the medical profession or married adults. Alfred Fournier's French Society for Sanitary and Moral Prophylaxis, for example, entitled their popular pamphlets *For Our Sons, When They Turn Eighteen* and *For Our Daughters, When Their Mothers Judge This Advice Necessary*, suggesting in the title that this material should be passed from doctors and parents to children only when they were ready for marriage and adult responsibility. The texts combined medical and social commentary, assuming that parents or even physicians would be guiding adolescents through material children could not access themselves.[9]

Progressive-Era writers and later scholars have often incorrectly assumed that information regarding sex did not exist. Birth control advocate Margaret Sanger, often prone to exaggerating her evidence to further her cause, wrote that there existed almost no information about sex in the early 1920s.[10] Perhaps her own run-ins with the 1873 Comstock Act, which reflected the Victorian code of silence, influenced her views. Yet she had been an active sex education lecturer among socialists and sex radicals in New York since at least 1911. She spoke at the Ferrer Center, an anarchist school for radicals, and the Heterodoxy feminist club in Greenwich Village. Thus she expanded her influence among Greenwich bohemians and free-love advocates.[11] In 1912 and 1913, Sanger wrote a series of sex education articles for the New York *Call*, entitled "What Every Girl Should Know," only to have Anthony Comstock ban it as obscene.[12] Educational material may have been hard to decipher or hard to procure for all but the literate elite, but, despite Comstock's vigilance, a significant literature on sex education existed since at least the nineteenth century.[13]

A robust sex advice and educational literature relied primarily on the work of clergy, doctors, and moral reformers, who tended to adhere to middle-class standards of propriety. They assumed, or wrote as if they assumed, that sexuality would be expressed only within the confines of marriage and would be used for only reproductive purposes. These books targeted white middle-class Americans as their audience.[14] Because publication of books and advice from private physicians was the foremost method of sex education, the material was largely limited to literate Americans wealthy enough to purchase books or pay a doctor.[15] Most writers advocated restraint as of the utmost importance to health and well-being, although some medical and lay advice countered with the ancient belief that continence was harmful to men.[16] Prominent health reformers like John Harvey Kellogg highlighted the health dangers of sexual indulgence, especially with prostitutes.[17] They also assumed that women had little interest in sex outside of procreation, whereas men had to fight off their natural sexual aggression to maintain notions of "civilized morality."[18] Sexual activity outside of marriage signified a failure to conform to middle-class ideals. Sexuality within marriage gained more opportunity for expression with the development of new and more effective forms of contraception and increased communication between partners about the desire to limit fertility. Moral reformers of the nineteenth century included those who rejected sexuality entirely, such as the Shakers. Other moral reform groups such as the Mormons and the Oneida Community experimented with new forms of extramarital or nonmonogamous sexuality. Debate over these groups' beliefs, and their beliefs in the connection of sexual behavior to physical and spiritual health, contributed to a greater dialogue on what defined sexual normality and expectation.[19]

The Progressive Era can be viewed as the culmination of a revolution in American attitudes toward sex.[20] In the first decade of the century, reformers attacked "two fundamentals of Victorian morality, the conspiracy of silence and the double standard."[21] They first had to fight the fallacy that ignorance was innocence, that children not instructed in sex education would neither have sexual thoughts nor participate in sexual activities. By the 1910s, Bigelow and others stressed that ignorance itself was nearly impossible: "It is usually an easy matter to protect children against smallpox and typhoid and some other diseases, but no parent or educator has yet found out how we may be sure to keep real live children ignorant of sex knowledge."[22] The debate should not be over the acquisition of knowledge but its source: "whether parents and trained teachers rather than playmates and other unreliable persons should be the instructors."[23] This was the mission of the new wave of sex education organizations. They believed that the home and the church had failed in their duties, and they wished to either assist or supplant the old institutions as the source of sexual information. Once this idea moved past mere purity to medical hygiene, the topic faced considerable controversy.

From Social Purity to Social Hygiene

The social hygiene movement developed out of a strain of purity activism of the late nineteenth century, which emerged from antebellum reform movements like women's rights and abolitionism.[24] Bringing together evangelical Christian strategies with interest in the uplift of all people, the purity movement had a national following by the 1880s. Originally founded by the Church of England in 1883, "White Cross" societies were quickly adopted by American Episcopalians to promote sexual purity among young men. White Cross societies, similar in design and organization to temperance societies, urged young men to take "the pledge" to stay pure until marriage, equating the poisoning influences of sex to those of alcohol or tobacco.[25] One form of the pledge, published in the *Philanthropist* read:

I, _____ Promise by the help of God.
   1. To treat all women with respect, and endeavor to protect them from wrong and degradation.

2. To endeavor to put down all indecent language and coarse jests.
3. To maintain the law of purity as equally binding upon men and women.
4. To endeavor to spread these principles among my companions, and to try and help my younger brothers.
5. To use every possible means to fulfill my command: "Keep thyself pure."[26]

These groups were decentralized, lacking formal documents or institutional records, but scholarly estimates place their memberships in the tens of thousands. Influence and visibility spread when the Woman's Christian Temperance Union (WCTU) adopted White Cross activities, dubbing purity work among girls "White Shield" societies. Even early in the movement, racial language linked whiteness with sexual purity. Likewise, Christian identification suggests anxiety about non-Christian (or even non-Protestant) members of the body politic bringing alternate moral codes to America through increased immigration in the late nineteenth century. Gendered language illustrates assumptions about male and female sexuality. The men's work stressed Christian morality and choice in its symbolism, while the work with girls stressed the need for a "shield" for protection.[27]

In an era when whiteness was not simply defined by skin color, white supremacists, associating whiteness with sexual purity, could easily reverse the formulation and assume nonwhite people to be sexually impure. Those wishing to achieve "whiteness" might attempt to do so by adopting the rhetoric and behaviors of respectable sexual Victorianism. Whiteness also connoted belonging in the national body politic, conveying political, social, and cultural benefits. New immigrants and those whose racial purity was in question had to prove their whiteness and their purity, often through adopting the cultural norms or ideals of the dominant group. To be white, one had to be pure. And vice versa.[28]

Purity advocates usually shrouded their messages in lofty euphemism.[29] Despite this unspecific language, they provided at least a modicum of sex education to male and female youths. The main group of purity advocates was the American Purity Alliance (APA), which consolidated in 1895, uniting many local moral education societies under the leadership of Aaron M. Powell. It built upon men's White Cross work and middle-class women's purity work with "fallen" women.

Under the umbrella organization formed by the APA, women activists targeted working-class girls, assuming they were in most need of protection or most likely to turn to prostitution. One contributor who advocated greater legal protection for girls wrote, "It is the young, ignorant, and inexperienced, who are most easily led astray, especially the children of pinching poverty and want."[30] Another noted that working-class girls, out from under their parents' watch at too young an age, needed an agency such as theirs to step in and teach them what their parents, through poverty or ignorance, failed to do. Here again, both cultural and biological assumptions shaped middle-class women's ideas about working-class girls. Protection of working girls involved both an assumption about the dangers poor girls faced and assumptions about their sexual precocity and moral degeneration.[31] Anna Rice Powell, wife of APA founder Aaron M. Powell, described the aims of the purity movement and sex education: "To give the girls some knowledge of their physical structure and the special functions of their sex, to teach them to reverence the body as the very temple of the Holy Spirit, and to deplore every thought, act, and habit that profanes it."[32]

Within the purity movement, dissent arose over the matter of race. Several African American purity activists decried the way the movement, and American society as a whole, did not offer the same protections to black women that they did to white. Writing in 1896, purity advocate Martha Schofield outlined how the institution of slavery permitted the sexual exploitation of black women and denied black men the right to protect them. Schofield concluded that the legacy of slavery hurt the purity of both races, as it taught blacks dangerous habits and taught whites to look down on blacks. She praised the WCTU for its efforts, but she pointedly noted the shortcomings of white purity workers who overlooked race: "Their work combined with the education efforts to lift colored women to a higher wifehood and holier motherhood is one of the means. The still greater need and only safe building for the future is to teach *boys*—yes, *boys*—the danger and the wrong, and lift men to the responsibility and nobleness of fatherhood and to respect *all* women." She showed frustration with the sexual double standard, society's failure to recognize men's responsibility in the downfall of women, and society's failure to include black women in the category of "*all* women."[33]

Schofield was not the only one who recognized the challenges of including all women in the purity movement. WCTU and National Association of Colored Women activist Frances E. W. Harper noted, "Friends, I need not tell you that I belong to a race which more than thirty years ago stood on the threshold of a new era. A homeless race to be gathered into homes, a legally unmarried race to be taught the sacredness of the marriage relation." Harper concurred with Schofield by stating that enslaved African Americans had been forced into impure sexual relations, but she then put the blame on white women who cared only "for the purity of her daughters and not her sons; for the purity of the young girl sheltered in the warm clasp of her arms, and not for the servant girl beneath the shadow of her home." Just as she had in the WCTU, Harper urged whites to consider gender and race when conducting purity work. "As crime has neither sex nor color, so its prevention and remedies should not be hampered by either race or sex limitations."[34] While only a small minority within the movement, black women provided a vocal critique of purity workers who too easily assumed that the womanhood they protected was always white.[35]

Besides the challenges of race, purity activists had to cope with strained relationships with the medical community. Many distrusted doctors who treated patients with venereal disease, arguing that such doctors enabled sin, prostitution, and the double standard that permitted male sexual indulgence. APA leader Aaron Powell attempted to bridge the gap, demonstrating that many physicians could be allies of the movement rather than enemies. Powell labored to obtain the signatures of physicians to support his "Medical Declaration on Chastity," which proclaimed "that chastity—a pure, continent life, for both sexes—is consonant with the best conditions of physical, mental, and moral health."[36] Now with alliances among some medical men and women, the APA worked in conjunction with the YMCA and other youth organizations to distribute purity literature in cities across the country. Under the leadership of Prince Morrow, suspicion between physicians and purity advocates began to fade.

Prince Morrow and ASHA

Dermatologist and syphilis expert Prince A. Morrow wished to further unite purity and medical hygiene groups to lay the groundwork for a unified sex education movement. Morrow represented a new wave among medical doctors, willing to challenge the conspiracy of silence that pervaded the medical profession. Despite the supposed shield of scientific disinterest, many physicians in the late nineteenth and early twentieth centuries hesitated to discuss sex or venereal disease for fear it would sully their reputations. Morrow, however, had translated the works of French dermatologist and venereal expert Jean Alfred Fournier in the 1880s and attended the first international conference on venereal diseases in 1899. In 1902, Morrow attended a second international conference in Brussels, Belgium, where he was asked to begin a society in the United States for the control of venereal diseases, similar to Fournier's French Society of Sanitary and Moral Prophylaxis. Participants set out to combat syphilis through a program including the suppression of prostitution, diagnosis and treatment, and widespread education on the subject.[37] An article Morrow published in 1901 discussed how the moral and medical communities should unite behind similar goals and efforts: "It is unfortunate that there should be such an irreconcilable conflict of opinion between the hygienist and the moralist upon this important question. The medical man and the moralist are both interested in the correction of the social evil. Instead of working independently, and often antagonistically, there should be cooperation and concert of action." Morrow blamed the antagonism on purity reformers who feared that information about treatment of VD would lead to greater promiscuity.[38]

As physicians expanded their understanding of venereal diseases, many doctors began questioning the accepted silence or resistance of their colleagues about such critical issues. Would they have to maintain the conspiracy of silence, when speaking out could actually help people lead healthier lives? In the early twentieth century, a few, led by Morrow, spoke out. Activist physicians formed social hygiene organizations associated with the AMA or local medical organizations, giving speeches to medical societies, schools, or women's clubs about the dangers of syphilis and gonorrhea.

Morrow chose to emphasize education to promote purity rather than to increase marital satisfaction. He argued that all possible social institutions, including the press and the schools, should share information with adults and children alike.[39] He argued that both physicians and purity reformers should stand against the conspiracy of silence and the double standard.[40] Until his death in 1913, Morrow worked tirelessly to gather supporters, study the problem, and devise solutions to social ills caused by extramarital sex and sexual ignorance.

Morrow believed success required two pillars: first, slowly changing public opinion to favor a general acknowledgment of sexual problems and, second, encouraging a concrete discussion of medical, social, and educational methods to alleviate those problems. Morrow linked the medical problem of venereal disease with the social concern that "deviant" sexual behavior would erode the very basis of American civilization.

Morrow outlined his social and medical justification for sex education in his book *Social Diseases and Marriage* (1904). He supplemented its medical basis with a righteous anger against the previously widely held belief that God sent venereal diseases to punish sinners. He wrote, "In the popular conception venereal diseases are diseases of debauchery—confined to an obnoxious class or their consorts—which carry with them the stamp of licentious living. They are without the pale of public sympathy and public protection, because they are considered the result of immoral relations which are voluntarily entered into."[41] Through his own experience and in talking with his peers, Morrow knew that thousands suffered from VD they had contracted "innocently," usually specifying women who caught it from their philandering husbands (a danger of the sexual double standard). He was increasingly angered at the medical profession's willingness to protect men's sexual prerogative rather than women's health, to the point of refusing to notify a woman of the disease she had contracted to cover up her husband's behavior.[42] What is more, he fumed that society could not expect the young and ignorant to understand how to avoid such sin and disease if nobody taught them about it. "Can the young who have been brought up in entire ignorance of such matters be said to voluntarily expose themselves to dangers which they may not even know exist? Is not society to blame for this faulty training, or, rather, absolute lack of training, which exposes them to these dangers?"[43]

Morrow's gradual approach to reform did not advocate educating girls, however. On this subject, he wrote, "While it is not contended that the exposure of existing evils should form a necessary part of the education of young women, yet they should know something of matters which so closely touch their health, domestic happiness, and the future of their children." Girls, as future wives and mothers, needed protection from suitors with venereal diseases. Morrow suggested that girls rely on their fathers to inspect suitors. He continued, "She should know that dissipated men do not make desirable husbands," but not necessarily the medical and social reasons behind "dissipation."[44] Morrow supported a single moral standard, that society hold men to the same standard as it held women, but his understanding of sexual equality did not include equal education for the sexes.[45] Throughout his work, he specified education for young men and boys, not for young people and children. Morrow pushed the boundaries beyond what was expected at the turn of the twentieth century, but he remained mired in certain gender assumptions. His reform impulse included reducing the strength of the sexual double standard, yet he still did not consider women to be moral actors who made their own sexual decisions. An end to the double standard would occur not through equal rights of the sexes but through pure, chivalrous men and protected women.

He was reformist in his aims to unite the medical and moral aspects of sex education. Morrow wanted to redefine VD as a contagion separate from sin. He still addressed the sin that perpetuated the contagion, but he believed it was vital to provide moral education in conjunction with sex instruction. The clergy, he thought, "may be justly criticized for their indisposition to touch upon social evil. . . . The clergy are too prone to accept the archaic theory of the moral etiology of venereal disease." Morrow was frustrated with moralists' assumption that venereal disease struck only the guilty. He even pointed out the unchristian tendency of many physicians to "shrink from all contact with this social leprosy."[46] Morrow embodied a new alliance between the medical man and the moralist to work together to correct the "social evil" and the resulting diseases springing from it.

Morrow used his connections within northeastern Progressive circles to begin organizing. In 1905, he called a meeting at the New York Academy of Medicine, speaking to a small audience of his peers about the links among venereal disease, public health, and social ills. He argued that physicians, not clergy, possessed the best training to solve them. He advocated education as the best solution to these social ills, noting that men's sexual ignorance made the problem worse rather than better.[47] This core group formed the Society for Sanitary and Moral Prophylaxis. From 1905 to 1910, state and local societies tackling topics related to social hygiene formed in churches, women's clubs, and medical associations. ASHA cofounder Dr. William Snow regarded this period as a time of "industrious tabulation of scientific and social data and pioneer experiments in organization."[48]

Using a popular Progressive strategy, Morrow continued to publicize the problem. One contemporary eulogist wrote of Morrow, "He opened the door of publicity and let in the light of knowledge upon the slimy and festering course of the venereal diseases in their ravaging march among the ignorant and innocent."[49] Morrow urged legislative action, broad educational efforts, and better treatment of infected patients. In 1906, he wrote, "Publicity has come to be accepted as a sort of panacea for all social ills. Recent developments have demonstrated its remarkable value in the correction of certain public, political and commercial evils, especially those which are based on mystery and secrecy."[50] Morrow considered himself a muckraker, a term coined during the Progressive Era to describe writers who publicized danger and corruption in society.[51] He used his writings to undermine what he saw as a corruption in the distribution of medical information. More knowledge would provide people the ability to seek healthy (or eugenically suitable) spouses and to reject patent medicines sold by "quacks." He used both Progressive language and medical analogies for the need to remove the stain of disease from society. Medically, he argued, "so long as this foul ulcer in the flank of society is covered up and concealed, it will continue to fester and to send its infection through every part of the social body. It must be exposed and laid bare in order to be cured."[52] In the language of Progressivism, he noted, "The muck is there and needs to be raked."[53]

Morrow argued that sexual hygiene protected the individual, the nation, and "the race." In the early twentieth century, many Progressives understood this as a reference to the growing eugenics movement. The first and most obvious threat to the race was how venereal diseases manifested themselves in the infertility of women. "It is . . . the destructive effect of gonorrhea upon the procreative function that I would especially emphasize. . . . [German physician Albert] Neisser contends that gonorrhea is a more potent factor in the depopulation of countries than syphilis even."[54] He linked VD's threat to women's fertility to a much larger threat to the nation or race in general. Race—defined as the American, white, or even human race—needed protection from the threat of depopulation. Morrow's ambiguous language belied the fact that his concern with race suicide, like many others' at the time, had as much to do with white supremacy and the fear of its decline as it did with patriotic fervor. Morrow associated the venereal peril with the peril of foreign-born elements in America: "when we consider the cosmopolitan character of the population of New York, the large foreign colonies of Bohemians, Italians, Russian and Polish Jews, many of whom bring their social vices and sordid, communistic modes of living, it is quite possible that Fournier's figures [for high rates of VD infection] . . . may apply to this city as well as Paris."[55] In Morrow's writings, venereal disease encompassed the threat of national depopulation, the threat of foreign-born elements, and the collapse of the "traditional" family. America seemed to be going the way of decadent, depopulating France. It was an infection of the pure from a foreign source.

Like his colleague Fournier in France, Morrow faced the general assumptions of many Americans that venereal diseases were problems of "the city"—and by extension the poor and immigrant populations. Fournier worked hard to prove that syphilis existed in the countryside as well as the city. Morrow rarely found an audience for his work outside of major population centers. One exception, however, was in Indiana. John N. Hurty, secretary of the Indiana State Board of Health, was an early correspondent of Morrow. Hurty not only embraced Morrow's educational aims, but exceeded them. However, Hurty's goal went beyond a concern for venereal education to his own pet project: eugenic legislation. In 1907, Hurty's work impelled Indiana to become the first state in the Union to pass a compulsory eugenic sterilization law. Hurty's efforts in Indiana were not aimed at providing people with the knowledge necessary to make healthy decisions but at limiting the reproductive choices of people whom Hurty defined as "unfit" to breed.[56] Reformers' intent to limit the numbers of undesirables and increase the number of desirables, as well as dividing the desirable from the undesirable, led to increased Progressive interest in both eugenics and immigration restriction.

After five years of developing local societies and building membership for their organizations, in 1910 Morrow and his allies formed the American Federation for Sex Hygiene (AFSH) in St. Louis. The national organization encompassed Morrow's Society for Sanitary and Moral Prophylaxis and specifically aimed at the medical concerns surrounding prostitution and venereal disease.[57] Morrow's death in 1913 predated the official establishment of the American Social Hygiene Association in 1914. His work to bring together purity and medical reformers culminated in the union of the American Vigilance Association (the purity arm) and the American Federation for Sex Hygiene (the medical arm) to form ASHA.[58] The purity journal *Vigilance* welcomed the merger, announcing that "its aim will be to join scientific knowledge and methods with moral enthusiasm in a forward movement which the present widespread interest in the problems of sex makes opportune."[59] It became the embodiment of Morrow's 1904 platform, "whatever may be said of the practical unwisdom of attempting to mix morals and medicine, it cannot be denied that in the causation of sexual vice two factors, one a physical and one an immoral impulse, are intimately involved."[60]

Incorporated in early 1914, ASHA adopted a strategy to promote sexual health and morality. First, its members aimed to study prostitution and the police response to it. Second, it advocated "effective police procedure and effective legislation with regard to vice." Third, it promoted "total abstinence, and the provision of wholesome pleasures, both out-of-doors and in-doors." ASHA endorsed the supposed links between sexual maladjustment and such habits as indulging in alcohol, tobacco, and hot spices and overeating. It urged a "wholesome" lifestyle, including exercise, fresh air, and a plain diet (harking back to John Harvey Kellogg) to decrease sexual appetite. ASHA pioneer Charles Eliot, the former president of Harvard University and an influential voice in educational reform, specified that the link between alcohol and prostitution was specific to the "white race" only. Apparently, Eliot assumed either that all nonwhites abused alcohol or that nonwhites were doomed to impurity from alcohol and sex. Under Eliot's leadership as cofounder and first president, ASHA focused its attention on educating and reforming whites. Finally, the group's biggest challenge would be to introduce educational changes for "parents, then teachers, then adolescents, and lastly children."[61]

ASHA knew its success would lie in a cautious approach. Some adherents, such as Denslow Lewis, may have viewed the broad extension of scientific sexual hygiene information to the public as the ideal solution, but the public's resistance to both the content and the intended audience proved too great. Too many parents feared that any mention of adolescent sexuality would only incite dangerous activity; to both clergy and parents, discussion of sexuality appeared to challenge accepted religious and social taboos. The executive committee outlined its intentions to avoid these pitfalls in its first annual report: "direct propaganda has been made in behalf of sex education for both adults and adolescents but with the constant stipulation that it should be conservatively given by well-trained instructors, the adequate training of parents for the better enlightenment of their children being especially recommended."[62] ASHA wished to devise a strategy to encourage greater knowledge without raising the ire of parents, churches, or schools. To accomplish this, the organization decided to find morally acceptable agents to actually distribute the material. ASHA would supply the curriculum to parents, doctors, or social clubs, who would then distribute the material to children and adolescents at their discretion.

ASHA had considerable backing in Boston and New York, with other strongholds of support in San Francisco and Chicago. Growth was unsteady and uneven; local societies flourished in larger cities in the Northeast while elsewhere it garnered less interest. This may have much to do with a general assumption that prostitution and venereal disease were specifically urban problems;[63] it also demonstrated a tendency of the organization to target and reach an affluent, white, educated population, a group they believed could understand the benefits of social hygiene. Regional disparities were apparent from the start. The first annual report specifically highlighted ASHA's failure to permeate the South: "in addition to the lines of work already begun, a Southern Division office should be established as soon as funds are available." Executive counsel James Bronson Reynolds took a trip across the South in April 1914, visiting seventeen cities in seven states. Texas and Alabama each formed state social hygiene societies, but other tangible results were not forthcoming. ASHA mentioned provisional plans for a Southern States Conference but did not follow up on that development.[64] The report does not provide a reason, but it could be that ASHA lacked the money or grassroots support in the region. Its members feared that in one area, at least, southern cities were falling behind their northern counterparts: the abolition of prostitution.[65] ASHA's failure to infiltrate the South was attributed to southern resistance to northern "meddling," but it perhaps also reflected the organization's medical beliefs about the deleterious effects of hot climates on people's bodies and souls. Many physicians thought that hot, humid climates contributed to early sexual maturation and increased sexual impulse.[66]

ASHA dedicated much of its effort and funds to work surrounding the Panama-Pacific International Exposition, held in San Francisco in 1915, in an effort to correct some of the organization's regional disparities. The exposition included exhibits on such topics as tropical diseases and race betterment, which overlapped with some of ASHA's interests.[67] Despite concern over funding for such an undertaking, the executive committee therefore decided to contribute an exhibit to the exposition.[68] "Intensive efforts of the Association in the south and far west, described in the first report, were shifted to the middle west and to California as the site of the Panama-Pacific International Exposition," including an exhibit at the exposition that was seen by an estimated hundred thousand people.[69] ASHA's exhibit consisted of "a series of fifty wall charts supplemented by models, pictures, and illustrated albums dealing with the medical, educational, religious, and legal phases of social hygiene."[70] Illustrations designed to capture the attention attracted visitors to the exhibit, and staff then could either provide literature or counseling on social hygiene. It also made ample use of new technologies to increase the appeal of the exhibit and compete with better-known organizations for attention. "In the afternoon short talks by well-known experts, with lantern slide and motion picture illustrations, will present in popular form the public health problems involved in various diseases, including syphilis and gonorrhea."[71]

ASHA was deeply ambivalent about the exposition. ASHA field secretary Thomas Eliot wrote, "Exactly the same factors which make it an educational agency of far-reaching influence in spreading useful information upon every conceivable phase of human progress, may make it an equally far-reaching agency for disseminating vice and immorality." ASHA feared that the exposition attracted economically vulnerable young women seeking employment, and immoral men might lure those women into prostitution or immorality. Likewise, the organization chastised the City of San Francisco for failing to clean up its red light district or enforce moral policing in its dance halls. San Francisco's city officials had already labeled the local Chinese population as a source of both disease and vice. Local health officials in California often attributed bad health and morality to Asian enclaves like San Francisco's Chinatown, and they failed to lay blame on whites who were supposedly seduced by foreign vice.[72] Because of these hazards, ASHA also conducted a campaign to ensure the moral and physical safety of visitors and job seekers. It worked to reduce prostitution and support Travelers' Aid groups who organized to meet unchaperoned girls, and it lobbied the exposition organizers to make sure that both amusements and concessions "will be of the highest character; clean, wholesome, and free from objectionable features."[73] ASHA's efforts complemented those of other groups interested in the maintenance of girls' purity, such as the Young Women's Christian Association (YWCA), the Travelers' Aid Society, and the National Florence Crittenden League.[74]

The Panama-Pacific Exposition provided a major venue for the new organization to reach the public. The exposition's emphasis on race betterment and scientific advances brought national attention to the very subjects ASHA wished to put before a wide audience. Not only that, but it placed concepts of race at the center of the debate over medicine, sex, and eugenics.[75] ASHA went to considerable expense to have an exhibit at the exposition, working hard to forge ties to the multitude of related organizations such as the US Public Health Service, the Woman's Christian Temperance Union, and the American Medical Association.

The creation of ASHA gave purity advocates and medical hygienists the opportunity to work together to promote their common goals: an end to VD and better information for the public. Yet the organization maintained many of the racial, class, and gender assumptions that had limited its predecessors. Prince Morrow's efforts to unite the purity arm and the medical arm of the movement had created a nominally national organization, but ASHA's real reach did not extend far beyond the white, middle-class, northeastern Progressive elite.

By 1915, ASHA feared not just the anti–sex education backlash but the dangers of financial extinction. Despite its active work in San Francisco and elsewhere, the executive committee feared that war in Europe, which erupted in August of 1914, might detract from its efforts. Long before an American declaration of war, philanthropists and reformers diverted attention from their domestic agenda into war relief. Membership continued to grow slowly and spread unevenly throughout the country. With its armies mustering, ASHA began talking strategy: How could it move beyond public resistance and educate the masses? The most obvious solution, moving social hygiene into the schools, created its own set of problems and its own opposition.

Chapter Two

Parental Prerogative and School-Based Sex Education

At the Fourth International Congress on School Hygiene in 1913, teachers and medical professionals came together to discuss the health and hygiene of schoolchildren, tackling topics like sanitation, contagious disease reporting, and the purity of fresh milk. However, gynecologist Robert Willson expressed his desire to move beyond health care in the schools and into social hygiene: "It seems a far cry to those of us who were at work in this field twenty years ago to the eager demand for sex instruction and sex knowledge that is heard to-day on every hand from the parents of children. A long hard road has been traveled, the first portion very steep and hazardous, the latter part so easy as almost to appear treacherous." Little did Willson know how prescient his statement was! The road ahead was indeed treacherous, as social hygienists, who had made deep inroads in the conspiracy of silence, faced new and greater challenges to establishing sex education curricula in the public schools. While many Americans were more accepting of sex in the press and in reform circles, most still were not willing to put it in schools. Willson seemed genuinely surprised that he and his fellow advocates would meet such resistance. Yet that is exactly what happened.[1]

When Willson spoke in 1913, the time seemed ripe for bringing sex to school. Progressive educators recognized that the schools provided merely one of many institutions for social education. Schools necessarily competed with the family, churches, civic organizations, and the state. Across the country, Progressives prompted the formation of institutions such as settlement houses to meet the changing needs of a modern, industrialized nation. Settlement houses provided a wedge to reach people in need, and reformers saw the broader public school system as the ideal habitat for an even larger program of community outreach, reform, and uplift. But during the early years of the twentieth century, public schools began taking over more and more educational responsibilities that had traditionally been in the domain of the home. This involved everything from adult education and citizenship classes for new immigrants to bathing students who did not meet the school's standards of hygiene. As one historian put it, "The syllabi said nothing about baths, and teachers themselves wondered whether bathing was their charge. But there were the children and there were the lice!"[2] Following the lead of settlement houses, urban schools hired nurses, installed showers, and educated their charges on proper hygiene and disease prevention.

Did the schools prepare students to face the new challenges of modern American life? Progressive educators hoped that innovations in the curriculum could supplement or replace the training students did not receive in the home. Some advocated including vocational training, moral instruction, English language classes, or training in health and sanitary practices. Once the schools were invested in bathing, grooming, and protecting their students' health and morals, it did not seem like a large leap to sex education. By 1913, parents and Progressives, clergy and the media were engaged in a heated debate over introducing sex education into the public schools. This chapter argues that social hygienists wanted to incorporate sex education into public school curricula but retreated from that stance because of parental and community resistance. The Chicago public school system's experiment with a Progressive social hygiene program demonstrated to the American Social Hygiene Association that public opinion did not favor a school curriculum in sex education. Instead, reformers had to develop new strategies to introduce the subject matter without threatening parental prerogative.

Progressive Education: Reform in the Schools

The philosophical origins of the American public school system, based on Horace Mann's nineteenth-century ideal that all Americans deserved schooling, promised great things in an era that linked knowledge with goodness and education with redemption. Like so many other reforms underway in the Progressive Era, the issue was complicated. School reform often divided between genuine efforts to uplift the citizenry and coercive attempts to stifle difference or deviance. Mann believed that the common schools should teach a consensus of social and political values. Schools provided a training ground to Americanize pupils.[3] How did Americans define that consensus? As the nation confronted widespread changes due to urbanization, industrialization, and increased immigration, the schools transformed into a much broader social institution and adapted to the heterogeneous population accordingly.

Owing to the needs of an increasingly pluralistic nation, with competing political factions divided by ethnic and religious ties, religion became one of the first battlegrounds. Mann's desire to spread moral standards in the schools could cause conflict between religion and morality. By the close of the nineteenth century, educator William T. Harris theorized that the school should pick up where outside institutions left off but must not trespass on matters explicitly the domain of other institutions. He approved of moral education but opposed religious education.[4] This distinction was hard for some to accept. Education reformer Charles Eliot feared for the future of American education in a place where cultural pluralism demanded a separation of religion and public schools. In a 1909 address, he said:

> It is almost impossible to separate morality from religion. You know our public schools have been forced by the very nature of our population, mixed as regards both race and religion, to abolish religious services within the schools. There is, therefore, no systematic or direct moral training in most of the public schools. This is the situation, an almost incomprehensible and wholly deplorable situation; for the schools are the chief hope of the country, as regards the preservation of our free institutions, and the uplifting of our extraordinarily heterogeneous population.[5]

Eliot, who supported expanded sex hygiene training in the schools, consistently linked morality with Christianity. He feared that any moral or sex education would be incomplete without religion. His unwillingness to separate morality and social hygiene from a specifically Christian mind-set belied discomfort with the presence of non-Christians in the United States in general, a problem that would recur in his work with the American Social Hygiene Association. In a 1914 article espousing sex education, he wrote, "Among contagious disease the most destructive to the white race are the diseases called venereal."[6] The next year, he noted, "If the civilization of the white race is to survive, it must be saved through the diffusion and adoption of sound policies in regard to social hygiene, carried enthusiastically and persistently into action."[7] Eliot's language demonstrated his concern with preserving the white race, his disinterest in nonwhites, and perhaps his assumption that nonwhites were doomed to suffer venereal disease whether or not they received education. Eliot was certainly not the only one preoccupied with white education. School segregation based on race solidified during Progressive era in the aftermath of the Supreme Court's 1896 *Plessy v. Ferguson* ruling upholding the constitutionality of racial segregation.[8]

School segregation was by no means merely a southern phenomenon nor one that merely drew lines between black and white. Booker T. Washington's Tuskegee Institute merely represented the most famous example of separate educational facilities (with separate curricula and goals) aimed at African Americans. California, for instance, long practiced segregating students by race. Local school boards drew lines between white Anglo and Mexican-American students. California senator James D. Phelan wrote positively about the state's efforts to segregate Japanese students from whites in 1906.[9] It was entirely within the Progressive ethos to encourage segregation as part of a scientific and efficient educational reform movement.

By the turn of the twentieth century, however, many Progressives embraced a broad belief that these other institutions were somehow failing much of the population. Schools, derided by muckrakers in the 1890s for being out of date and ill suited to modern life, needed to reform their mission and their place in society.[10]

High schools expanded dramatically during the early twentieth century. In 1900, only 10 percent of Americans age fourteen to seventeen were enrolled in a high school and only 8 percent graduated. By 1920, the graduation rate more than doubled to 17 percent.[11] Not only had enrollments increased substantially in high schools, but the national view of the high school's mission had expanded as well. The National Education Association's Commission on the Reorganization of Secondary Education listed seven "main objectives" of American secondary education, including health, citizenship, worthy use of leisure, and the development of ethical character.[12]

Progressive educators encouraged schools to adopt extracurricular subjects such as music, art, and foreign languages, as well as citizenship and moral training. Concurrently, conservatives who opposed the Progressive educational movement belittled new curriculum additions as "fads and frills," fashionable but unnecessary distractions from the basic curriculum. The resistance was especially strong when Progressive groups lobbied to increase educational opportunities for racial minorities. Secondary education for southern blacks, for instance, did not keep pace with the expansion of white schools. When black secondary schools existed, they often relied on white philanthropy, which often demanded a focus on vocational or industrial education in order to receive funding and public support.[13] That said, the divide between industrial education and liberal education was not as pronounced as white philanthropists have assumed. The model of industrial education espoused by Booker T. Washington often provided a considerable curriculum intended to foster industriousness and character development in black youth, much like that celebrated in white Progressive schools.[14]

The social hygiene movement gained momentum at the same moment that public secondary schools expanded their enrollments, their curricula, and their role in the social life of the community. With the added emphasis on health and sanitation, social hygiene education seemed a logical extension. ASHA and its predecessor organizations believed that in an ideal society, sex education would be addressed in an ethical, scientific manner in the schools, providing future generations with a thorough grounding in the subject. School reform during the Progressive Era pushed the public schools closer to the ideal, but there was still a long way to go.

Sex in the Schools

Despite its belief in the desirability of a comprehensive school program of sex education, ASHA avoided pushing a sex education curriculum in the public schools before World War I. Extrapolating from the reaction of parents and the medical community to its early efforts, ASHA rightly assumed that it needed to orchestrate a campaign to shift public opinion before any lasting change could occur in the schools. Without parents on its side, ASHA understood, the project would fail. The organization worked diligently to expand and shape the debate over sex education, thus contributing to the destruction of the conspiracy of silence.[15]

The American Federation for Sex Hygiene and its successor, ASHA, addressed some of the immediate concerns with social hygiene courses in the school in the early 1910s. ASHA disapproved of addressing sex education in a coeducational setting, fearing that the subject coupled with the proximity of male and female students would incite precocious and dangerous thoughts. Students, ASHA argued, would not feel comfortable asking questions in a coeducational setting, or even of a teacher of the opposite sex. Typical of Progressive reformers who embraced the cult of expertise, it also feared that public school teachers lacked competence.

Progressives wanted to guarantee that whoever taught these courses had the appropriate training and expertise. Coming at a time when educators faced repeated criticisms of insufficient training, reliance on outdated pedagogical tactics, and unwillingness to address controversial questions, this raised the hackles of many teachers. Like physicians, elementary and secondary educators were in the midst of their own movement toward professionalization, trying to move beyond the stereotypes of inept machine-politics appointees of the city or provincial schoolmarms of the countryside.[16] The field was also divided by gender, as the split between the mostly male administrators and the mostly female classroom teachers widened gaps in status and pay. The cauldron already was boiling when the social hygienists argued that teachers were unsuited to take on sex education.

Many social hygienists endorsed what they considered a simple solution: guest lectures by physicians. But this solution created another problem. Educators balked at the suggestion, fearing that "special" lectures would draw too much attention to a topic that they wished to make as inconspicuous as possible. Many reformers also feared that not enough female physicians would be available to lecture to girls. Ideally, Progressives wanted sex education to be seen as part and parcel of a broader curriculum in anatomy, health, morality, and sanitation. Classroom teachers would subtly integrate the material within existing biology courses and elsewhere where the material complemented and expanded on students' basic education. However, training teachers in sex hygiene through normal school instruction would take a long time. Those who supported sex education in the schools endorsed first approaching teaching colleges with the material.[17] The American Federation for Sex Hygiene's 1912 survey supported training in teachers' colleges, and Columbia University's Teachers College began a program to instruct future teachers on the subject matter and methodology to teach sex education. In 1914, Teachers College began its lecture series under the direction of biology professor Maurice Bigelow. "We cannot make permanent progress by emphasizing the need of sex-education unless we can give assurance that qualified teachers are available." Bigelow argued that without "safe and sure" instructors, armed with both the moral and scientific wherewithal to tackle the material, sex education in the schools would draw the ire of opponents and do more harm than good.[18]

The Opposition

Three main groups opposed sex education programs in the early years: social radicals, who opposed the moralistic approach; social conservatives, who considered it not moralistic enough; and a third group of opponents, who supported sex education but only outside the schools.[19] First, a small group of social radicals thought that ASHA and its predecessors presented sex in entirely too didactic terms. Medical journal editor William Robinson disagreed strongly with the approach of the AFSH. In 1910, he replied to a plea for support from the American Society for Sanitary and Moral Prophylaxis, decrying what he considered to be its unhealthy attitude toward sex:

> I shall not argue with you or attempt to convince you, as you would probably not understand me. You speak the language of the tenth Century; I speak the language of the 20th, or perhaps rather the 25th. You speak the language of gloom and reaction; I speak the language of joy and progress. You speak the language of the shackled theologian; I speak the language of the free scientist.[20]

Robinson approved of greater access to scientific sexual information in order to free society from artificial moral restrictions, and he saw the society's approach as merely reinforcing those restrictions. Robinson published his own sex education treatise in 1916, in which he prescribed sexual activity to prevent mental sluggishness and impotence: "the exercise of the sex function is not a vital function; life does not depend upon it; but a person's all round physical and mental welfare does." He recommended condoms and other contraceptives for couples engaging in premarital sex. He advised men to not have sex with "any woman whom you do not know to be free from disease," but if a man could not help it, he should use a prophylactic. At the heart of Robinson's argument was that false religious and health consequences should not be used to scare people away from sex. He scoffed at the high venereal disease rates put forward by other writers and denied the legitimacy of any religious admonition to avoid sex. Robinson summarized that his program of sex education, unlike those put forth by ASHA and the purity organizations, "benefits everybody and it hurts nobody."[21] Robinson's critique rang true among the bohemian set of radicals who challenged "bourgeois" sexual morality and others who wished to separate sex from procreation, which included the burgeoning birth control movement of the time. This small faction urged a more sex-positive message in its efforts to prevent disease and sexual maladjustment.[22]

A second and much larger group worried that the opposite was true: that sex education in the schools would not adhere to accepted sexual moral standards. Some feared that the very discussion of the topic would lead to increased sexual activity among children and that teaching ways to avoid disease would only foster immorality. Dr. Richard C. Cabot explained, "Although doctors and parents should know about these matters, they shouldn't spin that knowledge out to children. The temptation to do this as a preventive measure is great, but the process is not wise. . . . It is the influence of pure personalities whom we mett [*sic*] that keeps us straight, not fear nor knowledge."[23] Catholic priest Richard H. Tierney, for example, attacked social hygiene proposals in the press. He wrote, "The more I ponder the means advocated to combat the social evil, the stronger grows my conviction that this whole movement will eventually fail of its high purpose." He criticized reformers' efforts to concentrate on science and intellect, arguing that knowledge would not contribute one whit to moral power. "The detailed teaching of sex hygiene,—especially if it be done through book and chart,—will make a strong impression on the young imagination. Sensuous images will crowd the faculty as bats crowd a deserted house. . . . Safety lies in diverting their attention from them." In fact, Tierney advocated diversionary tactics for children and adults alike. Ironically, his ideas were not as far as he assumed from the ideas advanced by the prohygiene forces, which also wished to prevent sexual activity through diversion. Several social hygienists argued that rather than pique interest in sex, a proper, scientific introduction to the subject would satisfy natural curiosity and prevent children's desire for experimentation.[24]

Tierney's apocalyptic imagery of falling dominos toppled by sex education in the schools read like the book of Revelations: "Two of the great natural protections of our children are modesty (reserve, if you will) and shame. . . . The public and frequent discussion of sex details will destroy both. Familiarity will breed carelessness. The lesson of the class will become the topic of conversation. Reserve will go. Shame will disappear. Sin will follow."[25] Tierney wanted not just to end social hygiene lessons but to excise all mention of sex from schools, novels, and theaters and to abolish dancing and coeducation after the onset of puberty.

Opposition to sex education expanded beyond the clergy and into the mainstream press. The popular magazine the *Century* also took a strong stand against sex education, as suggested by articles such as "The New Game of Playing with Fire and the Right Not to Be Forced to Know Evil." The article argued, "All over the country thoughtful parents are coming to the conclusion that it is neither wholesome nor necessary that the minds of young people should be constantly occupied with the public discussion of eugenics and the social evil. These are problems for adults, and require the most careful, discriminating, expert scientific study."[26] The American Federation for Sex Hygiene's 1912 survey uncovered several educators who remained hostile to the whole project. When asked at what age sex education should be introduced, H. H. Wilder of Smith College responded that he "would rather the children had no sex as long as possible."[27] Wilder's phrase notes a preference for "no sex," rather than no sex education. It is possibly a typographical error or misquote, but a telling one. It shows a conflation between the introduction of sex education and sexual activity, an assumption held by many who opposed social hygiene. While most critics did not agree with Tierney's extreme suggestions, many parents, educators, and politicians agreed with his basic argument: sex education was a morally ambiguous, if not dangerous, endeavor.

Besides those who opposed sex education on moral grounds, a third group endorsed the subject matter but feared that the public schools were absolutely the wrong forum. This third group stressed that the family, first and foremost, ought to introduce the topic. Reformers needed to avoid looking like they were coercing parents who did not wish their children to hear the lesson. Parents, critics argued, could best determine both the proper time and detail supplied to their children. Furthermore, parents could rely on the clergy and private physicians to supplement both the moral and medical sides of the subject, all in a context that was familiar, safe, and comfortable for the child. The heterogeneous population of the public schools augmented parents' fears. Ira Wile, a New York physician, agreed with the goals of ASHA, but he doubted the schools could provide the sort of education desired. "Here, then, is a teacher with forty children in a room, twelve to sixteen years of age, French, German, Italian, rich and poor, stupid and bright, sexually precocious and sexually immature—could that teacher teach them as a class group?"[28] Tellingly, Wile included the mix of sexually precocious and sexually immature, reflecting the difference in ages in various classes as well as the fear native-born, middle-class whites had of those they considered racially, ethnically or socially inferior.

Placing sex education in the schools raised the stakes over racial segregation in the schools. White San Franciscans challenged school integration in the 1900s by arguing that it would place white girls in close proximity to older Japanese boys, who were seen as a sexual threat.[29] Public health officials in Los Angeles racialized diseases, arguing whites who came into close social contact with Asians risked infection by germs and by bad manners and morals.[30] Wile shared the Progressive belief that a child-centered education could adapt to the needs of individual students, but even he thought that the schools had grown to the point that they could no longer safely perform this task. Different social groups distrusted schools for different reasons: for creating a venue for social mixing, for threatening parental prerogative and patriarchy, or for disrupting ethnic and cultural traditions.[31]

Besides the ideology of gender separation in schools, some reformers adopted very pragmatic challenges to high school sex education. AFSH survey respondents from all over the country wanted the subject to be introduced before high school, arguing that high schools did not reach enough people. For example, an educator at the New Jersey State Normal School remarked, "The teaching is needed in grammar grades as many children never reach the high school," a sentiment expressed by several others in the report.[32] The executive committee's report concluded, "Since numerous pupils never reach the high school, there is need of some definitely organized instruction relating to human life for pupils of grammer [sic] school ages. This is the most difficult problem now apparent."[33]

Besides the dropout rate by the time students reach high school, regional differences contributed to uneven enrollments. Geographic and economic limitations created a divide in student access among northern and urban schooling and rural and southern or western schooling.[34] Just as national organizations like ASHA lacked an even distribution of members and programs, so the American system of public education was not truly national. What is more, even if a district, city, state, or the nation could decide on a particular curriculum, its implementation would vary widely depending on individual teachers and school attendance.

Three specific factors contributed to the lag in education in the American South.[35] First, despite compulsory education laws in the early twentieth century, expansion of public school enrollments did not reach this still largely rural and economically poorer region as widely as it did in the North.[36] Much has been written about northern versus southern and urban versus rural school attendance rates. While the South appeared to have higher rates of enrollment than the North, southern daily attendance rates varied more depending on children's seasonal work commitments.[37] Racial and economic factors reinforced the lack of a uniform curriculum in rural America and particularly the South, especially considering the shortened school year and poor public support provided for African American schools. Even when enrollment did rise, many children of agricultural workers left school during busy seasons to help their families. Various "fads and frills" received even less public support in rural school districts. Even idealistic educators admitted that concentration on the basics was all they could accomplish with their limited resources, and supporters of educational retrenchment thought that additional topics would waste time and money or somehow render students unfit for their eventual positions in life.[38] White employers distrusted Progressive efforts to provide African American students with a liberal education, arguing that better-educated children would be less satisfied with their limited job prospects as sharecroppers or domestic servants.

Second, the prominence of evangelical Christianity in the South presented an obstacle to public discussion of sexuality and sexual development.

Evangelical religion played a crucial part in a more famous southern school debate in 1925, when the *Scopes* trial pitted evolutionism against biblical creationism in Tennessee public schools. Sex education, although not calling into question biblical literalism, brought to the fore similar questions about the interplay of science and values. Was the role of moral education in the schools changing? Was there a uniform method of teaching values to adolescents? How did scientific knowledge challenge traditional sources of expertise?

Third, a southern tradition of local control worked against any efforts, especially by national agencies or the federal bureaucracy, at implementing a far-reaching program for social hygiene or sex education. Historians of medicine have noted the difficulties outside "experts" faced in bringing new ideas or treatments to what they considered a blighted southern environment. Philanthropic organizations like the Rockefeller Foundation, in their attempts to rid the South of hookworm, met intense local resistance. Some local opponents went so far as to argue speciously that Rockefeller merely invented the hookworm scare as a way to sell shoes across the South.[39] Local control influenced the development of public schools and encouraged a reliance on parent- or church-centered education for southern children. Similarly, white southerners resisted northern involvement in the education of southern African Americans since Reconstruction, arguing that only southerners could properly understand and solve the problems of their local population.

Multifaceted resistance, coupled with broad regional differences, made the schools an unlikely home for sex education in the years before World War I. Where it was attempted, in northern, urban centers like Chicago, the results were less than promising.

The Chicago Experiment

In 1913, as the American Social Hygiene Association emerged from the union of the purity and hygiene movements, Chicago schools superintendent Ella Flagg Young took a bold step. She was the first woman to head a large urban school system in the United States and the first to implement a major sex education program in the public schools. Referred to as the "Chicago experiment," Young's program pushed through a new addition to the curriculum: three lectures for high school boys and girls on physiology, sexual morality, and venereal disease, to be presented by visiting physicians. Young and allies such as the Chicago Vice Commission and the Chicago Woman's Club researched and decried the increase in urban sexual danger, especially prostitution and venereal disease. Young's goal was to combat the rising tide of sexual immorality and venereal disease associated with the cities in the early twentieth century.[40]

Hoping the material would "get by" more easily, Young ordered the lectures to be presented to parents in order to gain their approval before the materials were introduced in the schools. The turnout was smaller than she anticipated, with only around sixty parents at each meeting. Public opinion still maintained that the family should be responsible for sex education. Apparently, things had not changed significantly since the 1899 Brussels conference on venereal disease, when the only concrete suggestion for public hygiene education for children was aimed at orphans who had no parents to fulfill that duty.[41]

Progressives doubted the effectiveness of teaching parents, despite the hope that doing so would reduce criticism that the schools were stepping in where they did not belong. According to Young, parents, the church, and the community were failing to educate their children on vital matters, and, even when they did, they lacked the necessary scientific expertise to do a thorough job. Progressive educators argued that many parents were already lost, exposed to years of poor habits and corrupting influences. The most efficient educational strategy was to reach children before they went bad, to mold them into pure citizens while they were still malleable. This was a common Progressive theory, pessimistically dismissing the past as lost while focusing on the perfection of the future through education of the next generation.[42]

Young believed the public schools had to overcome major drawbacks for social hygiene education to flourish there. She worried that some "precocious" children might be exposed to corrupting influences before they reached high school age. Young therefore advocated including "personal purity" talks aimed at elementary and middle school students to complement the high school curriculum. Better, she thought, to receive the correct information from the schools than incorrect and harmful information from the streets or peers.

High school students generally responded positively to Young's program, but the Chicago sex education experiment did not survive the academic year. Surveys demonstrated that an overwhelming majority of students favored including social hygiene in the regular curriculum. Parents had the option to withdraw their children from the special lectures, but few exercised the option.[43] While most students approved and most parents did not object, a few became openly hostile.

Pressure from school board members and protests from parents and local Catholic leaders forced Young to cancel the program. While the experiment predated the bulk of the Great Migration of African Americans to Chicago after 1915, Chicago certainly had a diverse population due to immigration. Polish, German, Irish, and Italian immigrants flocked to the city in the late nineteenth and early twentieth centuries, creating powerful ethnic enclaves and cultures. The weekly Catholic publication, the *New World*, denounced the experiment as "injurious to public morals," specifically Catholic morals.[44] Catholic fraternal organizations called upon the hierarchy of the Catholic Church to challenge new and dangerous innovations and presented a strong political threat in the machine politics of urban Chicago. Young's opponents threatened continued resistance to all of Young's Progressive endeavors if she did not halt the sex education program. They saw Young as the personification of Progressive interference in the private sphere. Parental prerogative trumped Young's vision for her schools.

Several of Young's strategic choices detracted from her ambitious aims. Most Progressive reformers, and indeed most ASHA members, thought that the Chicago program had flaws both in its planning and its implementation. Historian Jeffrey Moran notes that the experiment was "a case study demonstrating how not to implement sex education." Her attempt to the garner media support attracted particular attention to the program, including harsh criticism. The conspiracy of silence could not so easily be destroyed, and parents reacted with hostility to accusations that they could not properly shape their children's moral future.[45] Aside from the media attention, some opposed the strategy of the lectures themselves. The use of "special lecturers," considered necessary since teachers were not prepared to teach the subject, divorced the material from the regular curriculum of health, biology, or sociology, thereby attracting even more attention. The Chicago community rejected continuation of the program. Progressives may have believed that a scientific, publicized school campaign was the best approach. Nonetheless, it proved impractical. Until public opinion shifted, efforts to put sex education in the schools were rare, and they were more successful when sly and unobtrusive. Some instructors in subjects such as biology, health, and hygiene incorporated limited lessons in human reproduction and the rudiments of sexual hygiene without labeling it "sex education."[46]

Many reformers, educators, and medical professionals took the failure in Chicago as proof that sex education, even if suitable in other settings, did not belong in the public schools. The place reformers considered sex education most needed—the dangerous, sinful city—was also the place that held the most heterogeneous racial, religious, and ethnic populations. Presenting a politically viable common morality in sex education seemed impossible. Parents and communities did not wish to leave all mention of morality outside the schools; during the same period that schools considered and rejected social hygiene curricula, many states mandated antialcohol and antinarcotic education.[47] Schools in the Progressive Era continued a long-standing tradition in American education of using schools as a forum for instilling moral values in its citizenry.[48] But they drew the line at sex. Many feared that any mention of the material would only heighten students' awareness of and interest in the subject. Perhaps the topic was best handled through less formal means.

Parental Prerogative and Informal Education

Without schools as the location for sex education programs, where could ASHA turn for a wedge into broader society and the all-important younger generation? Its report on curriculum recommendations concluded, "The introduction of sex-instruction into the public educational system should be made carefully and with due regard to local conditions, such as the attitude of school officials, public opinion, and the availability of specially trained teachers."[49] Between the lines, both those who supported sex education and those who opposed it expressed concern about their ability to provide practical sex education for nonwhite, non-native-born, and non-middle-class populations. ASHA believed these groups were most in need of attention, but they were also the most difficult to reach and possibly the least likely to benefit from a sustained effort. If the contours of regional economy, politics, and culture pushed sex education away from the schools, what were the alternate paths? Would they differ based on race, gender, and class? Ever cautious of their public image and not wishing to be rejected entirely, many reformers took smaller steps to gain the public's approval or to find less noxious ways to introduce the topic to parents and children alike.

Despite the reservations held by some Progressives who adhered to the cult of expertise, most Americans still looked to parents as the most appropriate and effective source of information for their children. The *New York Times* reported in 1913 that the president of the New Jersey District Board of Education advised schools not to endorse sex education. "He held that educational leaders were making a mistake in trying to relieve parents of this responsibility," noting that the subject was best handled at home.[50] A more balanced response came from the *Journal of Education*, which stated, "Public opinion sharply voiced in many communities . . . is calling attention to the harm sure to follow the average schoolroom handling of the delicate topics involved. . . . The far-sighted reformer in matters of sex will think twice before asking the school to undertake indiscriminately and in mass what even fathers and mother, pastors and family physicians find it hard to do wisely for the children one by one."[51] Hard-liners and more tentative opponents agreed that other sources besides the school could provide the best sex education.

The American Society of Sanitary and Moral Prophylaxis kept in mind the importance of parental prerogative. Not wishing to rock the boat, in 1912 the society advocated educating mothers, allowing the mothers to pass information on to their children at their discretion. ASHA's education committee concluded, "It seems best to continue instruction to the mothers of children . . . but not to the children themselves at the present time."[52] They thought that interposing mothers was a necessary step toward a more complete education and a way to arouse less criticism from the general public. In the popular imagination, mothers embodied the benefits of women's supposed purity, plus the knowledge that came from marital and reproductive experience. The ASHA report showed that many leading educators endorsed this tactic: C. H. Levermore from Adelphi College favored "an attempt of the Public Schools to gather together the mothers and give them proper instruction." Another respondent suggested talks should be given to mothers with their daughters and father with their sons. C. W. Fowler of the Kentucky Military Institute suggested that "parents must be aroused by a meeting at the school house social centers where plain talks are given them to be passed by them to their children"[53]

ASHA incorporated this approach in its work at the 1915 Panama-Pacific International Exposition. Field secretary Thomas Eliot described a "common and largely justifiable popular prejudice against 'introducing sex instruction into the schools,'" and suggested pulling aside parents as well.[54] Harking back to Fournier's earliest books on sex education, the exhibit concentrated on providing educational materials to parents. "Several children have been instructed in company with their parents with charming results." ASHA offered personal counselors, available for appointments with parents to teach them how to instruct their children.[55] Having experts train parents could expand sex education without threatening the quality of the curriculum or the moral and religious objections of the family.

Educators had debated parental interposition well before the Chicago experiment. Unitarian minister Edward Griggs stressed the need of parents and teachers to work together in his 1903 monograph, *Moral Education*: "the great need, therefore, is that parents, teachers, and all concerned in the moral education of children should undertake the task of giving the needed information, while maintaining a reverence for the native veil of modesty that should always clothe this aspect of life."[56] He suggested an ideal solution in which parents laid out "a long period of quiet preparation" to be followed by teachers' "period of action." Griggs was quick to point out the danger in trying to completely deny the existence of sexual need. His vaguely anti-Catholic rhetoric noted that sex (within marriage) should not be "in itself evil" or "a sanctioned indulgence of human weakness." This teaching, he believed, prevented children from growing up to form healthy families. The ultimate goal was to avoid precocious stimulation of interest in sexuality. And Griggs, like so many others, advocated a vigorous outdoor life to distract children from their awakening desires.[57]

Interposing parents between educators and children gained approval on both sides of the Atlantic. Like Griggs, British educator Edward Lyttleton feared that if public schools were to incorporate sex education into their curriculum, it would eliminate two traditional influences: family and religion. In 1913 he wrote, "The first step to take is for clergymen and schoolmasters to insist in season and out of season on the obligation resting on parents not to leave this particular sort of instruction out of account in the training of their children." Lyttleton suggested that parents could and should turn to teachers and ministers to gather information but that they must be the ones to communicate those ideas to their children.[58] "Every possible effort should be made to induce the parents to undertake the task."[59] However, Lyttleton ended his article with a note of pessimism: "I am convinced that nothing will make either the parents or an adequate number of teachers grapple with this and similar questions with single mindedness, hope, and spiritual power, except a deeper and more widespread implanting of the truths of the Christian Gospel."[60] Lyttleton framed the crisis in terms not of state intervention but of the importance of a return to the church.

For the time being, ASHA capitalized on the benefits of working outside the schools. Morrow and his associates' pragmatism trumped idealism. Even before the failure in Chicago, public schools seemed a less than optimal location for sex education. As early as 1909, Morrow expressed a desire to introduce social hygiene into the colleges by forming alliances with college presidents, "but unfortunately very few of these college presidents are of President Eliot's way of thinking." A more practical alternative seemed to be forsaking the school and focusing on institutions more willing to endorse the cause. "It was suggested that possibly this work could be best accomplished through the agency of the Students Y. M. C. Association, a branch of which I am told exists in every college in the country." Morrow recognized the benefits of a "very close affiliation" with the YMCA and wished to capitalize on that, at least until schools could be convinced. That would take time.[61]

Morrow's turn toward the YMCA revealed a new strategy to keep sex education in the voluntary realm. In the American Federation for Sex Hygiene's 1912 survey, numerous educators from all regions of the nation who supported sex education in the schools also expressed the opinion that voluntary clubs and associations might provide a safer path. One professor at the University of Chicago believed that "in addition to schools and colleges, Churches, Sunday Schools and Clubs can help in the teaching." A respondent from Philadelphia replied, "Clubs, Sunday Schools, and Girls' Friendly Societies can be of help." A. H. Wilde of the University of Arizona suggested that clubs could fill the gap for pupils who did not attend high school. Samuel Lee Hornbeak of Trinity University in Texas wrote, "Most parents will not give the needed instruction," suggesting that clubs or organizations send lecturers from place to place to pick up the slack.[62] After the failure of the Chicago school program, many social hygiene reformers saw these alternate venues as more suitable and successful locations for sex education than the public schools.

As the Chicago experiment demonstrated, the public was not ready to embrace a forthright campaign for sex education in the schools in 1913. Therefore, ASHA sought to forge ties with some of the most reputable organizations of the time. It also recognized the practical importance of respecting family and religious spheres of influence. In 1914, the executive committee announced, "For the present, the Association hopes to do the greatest part of its educational work through other organizations—such as men's clubs, women's clubs, Young Men's and Young Women's Christian Associations, granges, benefit societies, state boards of health . . . and medical societies."[63] By working through other organizations, ASHA could reach a wider audience and shield itself from criticism if the organizations overstepped their bounds. Its goal of broadening knowledge of social hygiene could be met through teachers, parents, clergy, or any person with the proper expertise and moral influence. Yet this strategy inherently changed the message. Sex education curricula, adopted by character-building youth organizations that flourished during the Progressive Era, would take on religious overtones and focus on the white male experience.

Chapter Three

Sex Education for Whites Only?

In the early years of the twentieth century, a young boy attending a YMCA sum- mer camp at Camp Kiamesha, New Jersey, approached his counselor with a guilty secret. He had been masturbating and feared both for his health and his soul. His counselor confessed that he, too, was unable to overcome the sin of masturbation. He recommended that the two pray together, hoping that God would relieve them of their sin. The camp counselor, eighteen or nine- teen years old at the time, would recall this incident as a formative memory of his youth, noting both the expected response from youth organizations such as the YMCA—prayer—and its failure to solve what he would later accept as natural sexual feelings. Finding his own early encounters with sex education inadequate and harmful, the counselor would later build a career and interna- tional reputation around sex education. He worked to create a broader scien- tific knowledge of sexuality, accept it as part of biological life, and break down the stigma surrounding it. His name was Alfred C. Kinsey.[1]

Kinsey's adolescence suggests how white middle-class youths in Progres- sive America found themselves at the center of a maelstrom of social concern. How would the young men of his generation cope with this crisis of manhood? Industrialization and urbanization threatened traditional definitions of man- hood, causing many Progressives to fear that the boys coming of age around the turn of the twentieth century would be soft, weak, or feminized.[2] President Theodore Roosevelt exaggerated the perception of a crisis in masculinity in order to offer his own brand of militarized masculinity. Roosevelt advocated the strenuous life for American boys: a combination of vigorous outdoor activ- ity, character training, and absolute sexual continence. Character building allowed American boys to strengthen their bodies and their morals. Through this regimen, Roosevelt believed boys would grow to be fine citizens and good soldiers, form strong families, and build an ascendant nation.[3] As always, the ideal and the reality were worlds apart.

What part did sex education play in the creation of a strong, masculine citizenry? Unlike the medical advocates who dominated the American Social Hygiene Association, many youth organizations that undertook the topic before World War I de-emphasized disease prevention in favor of morality training in order to "build character" among those they wished to educate. They taught social hygiene by stressing religion, character, and chivalry rather than (or accompanying a tiny dose of) medical or biological sex information. Sex education helped form the identity of white middle-class boys by separating them from girls, from the poor, and from their nonwhite counterparts.

This chapter looks at the creation of adolescence in America and its impact on the sex education movement. Several influential organizations such as the Young Men's Christian Association and the Boy Scouts of American attempted to address the issue of sex education, although not all actually provided sex education. Their affiliated women's organizations took a less vocal stance on the issue owing to assumptions about middle-class white girls' adolescence and sexual development. White middle-class concepts shaped these groups' strategies. They created programs centered on morality, chivalry, and character development to build a class, gender, and race-based ideal of adolescence.

The Invention of Adolescence

Recent scholarship has placed sex education in the context of the history of education and gender, but few scholars have examined the place of class and race.[4] Historian Jeffrey Moran uses G. Stanley Hall's psychological and sociological model of adolescence as a framing device that creates a clear narrative for white middle-class youth but does not necessarily apply to a wider population in the early twentieth century.[5] Later chapters of this book will examine the different strategies used to address alternative audiences, such as African Americans. For now, let us look more closely at why Hall's theory of adolescence was racially specific.

G. Stanley Hall, first president of the American Psychological Association, published his two-volume study, *Adolescence: Its Psychology and Its Relations to Physiology, Anthropology, Sociology, Sex, Crime, Religion, and Education*, in 1904. Hall popularized the idea that adolescence was a distinct stage of life. Physicians and laypeople of course recognized many of the outward signs of puberty, but they rarely connected them to psychological and social changes that formed the basis of "adolescence." Teenagers, Hall argued, went through a period of intense "storm and stress" while they mentally, physically, and emotionally developed into adulthood. Some scholars argue that Hall's work invented, rather than discovered, adolescence. It was a new definition given to an expanding liminal period when youths were no longer children but not yet adults.[6]

The storm and stress of adolescence, as Hall described, held meaning only for a specific class and race in turn-of-the-century America. The hallmarks of adolescence—prolonged schooling and a debate over career aspirations—did not fit the experience of either racial minorities or the working class.[7] Only the white middle and upper classes had the economic wherewithal to maintain their children through high school or beyond and allow children the choice of numerous professions. The black children of sharecroppers who attended schools only in winter or dropped out to work full-time by the age of twelve certainly did not experience this version of adolescence.[8] Hall's description set males as the norm and relegated the female experience to the sidelines, an issue that is discussed later in this chapter. Hall's northeastern assumptions also took regional differences for granted. Access to schooling did not keep pace with compulsory education laws of the late nineteenth century, especially in the South, the West, and in rural areas. High schools particularly were concentrated in the more urban northeastern United States.

According to Hall, white adolescents experienced the physical changes of puberty as they simultaneously gained a wider receptivity to the emotional and spiritual world. They were more prone to religious conversion, to deliberations of higher ideals and morality, and to a romantic idealization of the chivalric days of the past. A flood of evangelical organizations emerged in the late nineteenth century, fearing that churches were losing their social power and hoping to steer young people toward the Christian lifestyle. Starting in the 1880s, youth were "suddenly being discovered by the churches," as religious organizations emphasized shaping and occupying the spare time of the young.[9]

Hall also embraced "recapitulation," then a popular anthropological theory. Recapitulation stated that, like cultures, people went through periods of evolutionary development. Children were like savages who would gradually develop both an adult body and adult civilization. Hence, adolescents were trapped somewhere between savagery and civilization. Theorists used the analogy of the Middle Ages to note adolescents' anthropological development.[10] Prior to the publication of *Adolescence*, Hall's early academic work was popularized by William Forbush, whose widely read treatise, *The Boy Problem*, made waves in 1901. Forbush built upon Hall's early writings and categorized adolescence as an age of "temporary insanity": when "passion is most active, ignorance most great and self-control most weak."[11]

These theories were rooted in white assumptions that Africans and African Americans lacked the potential for fully developed "civilization." Recapitulation disqualified young blacks from experiencing the same mental and emotional development during puberty since they were purportedly centuries behind the white evolutionary experience. Forbush stressed that whites and nonwhites experienced puberty differently. "Racial differences are quite marked," with boys of a "tropical temperament" reaching sexual maturity at an earlier age than whites. Forbush, like other theorists at the turn of the century, did not see race as a black-white dichotomy. Influenced by the debate over immigration restriction permeating American society at the turn of the century, he described Irish, French-Canadian, and "Jew type" boys as racially different from the old-stock Anglo-Saxon white population. Forbush concluded that their ethnic heritage influenced their sexual development and their purported inclination toward antisocial and criminal behavior.[12]

A variety of organizations geared toward nurturing youth as they passed through the tricky teen years capitalized on these theories and contributed to the social hygiene movement. Groups like the Boy Scouts and the YMCA, as well as local civic or religious clubs, tied together adolescent development, character building, and sex education in an effort to inculcate moral purity, character, and white middle-class standards for adolescents. Forbush advocated organizing boys separately from girls and giving them steady physical activity in a country setting away from the dangers of the city. He equated urban life with sexual danger and promoted Progressives' efforts to reintroduce urban children to country living. He advocated sex-segregated, Christian clubs, camps, and recreational organizations, a popular concept that flourished during the Progressive Era.

The Bible as Textbook

Nondenominational groups like the YMCA and, to a lesser extent, the Boy Scouts of America, stressed the importance of inculcating religious ideals as they taught sex education. At the time, this was not considered unusual. Many people who discussed their early sex education mentioned the centrality of the Bible as a text. For example, the first known survey of the sexual knowledge and behaviors of American women, produced by Clelia Duel Mosher, noted that many women who had received little or no instruction from their parents turned to books, including the Bible, for their information.[13] Mosher interviewed 45 well-educated "Victorian" women. A more substantial sex survey, conducted by Katherine Bement Davis in the 1920s, included the responses of 2200 women. Davis reaffirmed Mosher's findings that young girls lacked adequate sexual information. Confused by their own bodies and the reticence of parents and teachers, girls furtively turned to books to answer their questions. Davis noted of one respondent, "From 15 years on she gained some knowledge of sex matters from 'a few dirty stories, the actions of my beaux, and the obscene portions of the Bible.'"[14] Davis's respondents turned to dictionaries, encyclopedias, and medical texts, as well as novels and other "dangerous" sources, to satisfy their curiosity. Another respondent's reply: "At about 11 years a schoolmate gave her a vague description of the sexual act. This aroused extreme curiosity—which she satisfied by studying the Bible, the dictionary, and a medical book called *The Cottage Physician*."[15] Access to professional medical books was limited, since many publishers labeled medical texts to be sold only to physicians and libraries kept them under lock and key.[16]

G. Stanley Hall imagined possible dangers inherent in using the Bible as a primary source of sex education. Hall consulted ophthalmologist Hermann Cohn, who worried that the Bible's more sensual passages led to masturbation, which Cohn believed contributed to eye diseases. Cohn advocated publishing a censored version of the Bible, one that omitted the reproductive and obstetric passages.[17] Hall also recounted an anecdote of a young man who lived in fear after his first nocturnal emission: "Bible passages greatly aggravated my fears, such as one in Deuteronomy XXIII [If there be among you any man, that is not clean by reason of uncleanness that chanceth him by night, then shall he go abroad out of the camp, he shall not come within the camp], and others; as I look back, my entire youth from six to eighteen was made miserable from lack of knowledge."[18] Hall understood that the Bible appealed to religious youths who lacked access to other sources of sex education, but he also recognized the possibility of misinterpretation and the Bible's shortcomings as a health-care text. Use of the Bible as a textbook—albeit an imperfect or incomplete one—for sex education continued, however, into the early decades of the twentieth century.[19] The Texas health guru, "Daddy" Flynn, hosted a series of lectures in San Antonio for men and women in which he stated "that the Bible was the greatest health book in the world."[20] He argued that the Bible taught a single standard of morality, respect for women, and respect for personal purity. Flynn's lectures demonstrated that the ties between sex education and religion remained strong into the twentieth century. Christian youth organizations like the YMCA built on these connections, incorporating morality as the cornerstone of healthy instruction in sex hygiene.

The YMCA

The YMCA was the most active youth organization of the era when it came to sex education. Originally formed in 1844 in London, its organizers designed the YMCA to cope with problems arising from rapid industrialization. First and foremost, the YMCA provided a place to stay for young men who flocked to cities in search of jobs. By 1851, the YMCA concept arrived in the United States, providing safe, inexpensive housing for working-class young men. Its stated purpose was to improve the spiritual, mental, social, and physical condition of young men. It arranged recreational activities and Bible studies to counter what the organization perceived as the dangers of city life: poor health and moral turpitude. By the 1880s, however, the aim and the clientele of the YMCA had shifted. More middle-class youths seeking work as white-collar clerks in the city utilized the YMCA as an institution of middle-class community building.[21]

The YMCA did not develop a systematic curriculum on sex education, but as a whole the organization approached the topic with zeal. The YMCA magazine *American Youth* dedicated an entire issue to sex education in 1913. It included articles by ASHA members Prince Morrow and Maurice Bigelow, encouraging broad educational programs. The YMCA encouraged pamphlets and lectures by physicians in the field and prided itself on providing practical, truthful, and uplifting information to young men.

George J. Fisher, a medical doctor and YMCA secretary, noted the organization's pioneering work and the unique traits that made it the ideal provider of sex education. The YMCA combined the positive elements of both school-based and home-based education, argued Fisher. "The people who should teach the subject are those in daily touch with the youth and not strangers, and those who do teach should be only those of unquestioned character and who stand in a position of leadership and respect to the youth and who teach them . . . with the social and moral emphasis." Parents and schoolteachers lacked the expertise; visiting lecturers lacked the camaraderie with the boys. Therefore, the YMCA representative was the ideal source of sex hygiene information: he was trusted and knowledgeable, had a rapport with the boys, and was of unimpeachable moral standing.[22]

Fisher also noted that the YMCA could develop lectures to suit diverse audiences. Not only did the YMCA segregate based on age, keeping boys from mingling with men, but it also provided different services for men of different classes and races. Black and white had been organized into separate chapters since the organization's inception. And after the 1860s secretaries began establishing chapters for specific immigrant and ethnic groups: German, Dutch, Chinese, and American Indian chapters formed to meet the particular needs of different groups and perhaps better teach them (white) American mores.[23] Likewise, sex education could be tailored to meet the needs of different groups. Fisher wrote, "Specific work is done for business men, railroad men, industrial workers, for men in the army and navy, for colored men, and for Indians. . . . These groups of men differ in the character of their needs, in the degree of their intelligence concerning the question, and in the intensity of their temptations. Consequently this segregation affords unusual opportunity for being specific in giving counsel."[24] This passage suggests that Fisher believed that a uniform curriculum was neither effective nor desirable in educational work but must be tailored to the stereotyped perceived needs of different audiences.

Fisher commended YMCA teachers, exemplified by Max J. Exner, who combined sex hygiene into a larger, and completely "natural and wholesome" approach to hygiene of the body, focusing on the "positive and moral side of the subject."[25] Max Exner, a physician and physical culture instructor, united his medical education and his passion for the YMCA health programs to introduce a sex education curriculum to YMCA boys wherever he could. Exner wrote, "The most effective sex education is that which is personal and individual, given in friendly heart to heart talks between adult—teacher or father—and boy."[26] He published numerous pamphlets for YMCA use on the topic but warned adults not to depend entirely on the written word: "literature necessarily lacks this personal element and, useful as it may be, it must not be relied upon too largely." He advised parents and secretaries to read the pamphlets and then communicate their content to the boys verbally, rather than giving boys the reading material directly.[27] Exner agreed with ASHA's assumption that reading materials might prove dangerous to young men if given without supervision.[28] Exner also stressed the importance of not allowing the topic to fall too far into discussion of pathology, as physicians tended to do, which would only serve to frighten and confuse laypeople.

The balance between religion and education was a tricky one for the YMCA. Exner warned against overt preaching, which was common among religious educators. YMCA administrators were particularly concerned about African American preachers (whom they dubbed "ranters"), stressing that schools in the black community might be a better way to reach the higher classes of blacks than churches, which ostensibly attracted not just the elite but also the uneducated masses.[29] Health workers at the YMCA, like Exner himself, could de-emphasize disease and focus on the religious ideals of sexual behavior, while not losing the boys' interest or the importance of scientific facts. It was a difficult line to walk, but Exner saw religion as the keystone. Echoing G. Stanley Hall's words, Exner noted that adolescent boys experienced the awakening of sexual desire at the same time as they experienced "love of God." If they could walk the fine line, the YMCA could effectively preach the word of God and teach hygiene at the same time.[30]

One YMCA secretary recorded in his memoirs both the benefits of the organization's sex education programs and the way race distorted them. Aaron G. Knebel grew up outside of Waco, Texas, at the end of the nineteenth century. His interests in gymnastics and Bible study eventually drew him into membership, and later a career, in the YMCA. Knebel recorded his surprise at the forthright attitude his local branch had toward sex education:

> Most boys of my acquaintanceship grew up in ignorance of matters related to sex life. Our parents did not discuss them with us. . . . It was not until I became a member of the Y.M.C.A. that I heard an adult, a fine Christian physician, tell a group of lads ranging in age from fourteen to sixteen about the reproductive organs. It was done so honestly and skillfully that it "registered." No longer were we ashamed of some things we had not heretofore understood.[31]

Knebel noted the problems the YMCA faced, especially in the South, in confronting such topics. During his tenure as a secretary in Charleston, South Carolina, Knebel confronted one of the young men in his program. "He had intimated in the presence of a small group that he did not believe it was a sin to have intercourse with a comely Negro woman."[32] Knebel was shocked because desires for interracial sex threatened white Christian men's ideas of sexual purity:

> In a perfectly candid manner [another] young man told me that when he reached his eighteenth birthday his father warned him never to take

advantage of a young woman of his race; to be a gentleman, to protect her by his chivalry. . . . Having given this admonition, he counseled him how to proceed when he reached an age or period in his life when the sexual impulse overmastered him. The father knew of several fine colored women whom the son might visit without fear of contracting disease.[33]

Horrified, Knebel took it upon himself, under the auspices of his YMCA work, to point out the shortcomings of the young man's argument. Christian character building was not primarily about preventing disease or, unfortunately, protecting black women, but about preserving men's purity and souls. However, when trying to open the conversation in his group Bible study, Knebel met with silence and resistance, likely due to his demand for an end to the racial and gender double standard.[34]

YMCA directors employed speakers and writers to work on their sex education campaign. Professor Winfield Scott Hall, a best-selling sex education author, toured YMCA facilities, high schools, and women's clubs preaching the importance of sex education. In 1910, he toured the Detroit area, working in conjunction with area physicians and educators.[35] His books advertised his service as a lecturer, with letters of reference from YMCA secretaries in Philadelphia and Chicago. Hall estimated in one advertisement that his lecture, "Sex Hygiene," was "heard by 50,000 men last year."[36] The organization's diverse educational and recreational programs made it a leading source of both character building and sex information in the early twentieth century. Yet its explicit Christian messaging alienated those outside the bounds of the dominant religion.

Alternatives to Christian Sex Education

In the early twentieth century, it was far more difficult to find character-building organizations adapted to non-Christians or even non-Protestants. The evangelical aim and the Bible-study basis of the YMCA alienated Jews and some Catholics from active participation. Alternate organizations, like the Young Men's Hebrew Association (YMHA) and local Jewish community centers, formed to provide similar support for Jewish immigrants in Baltimore, New York, and a few other American cities. Like the YMCA, the YMHA provided English classes, physical fitness activities, and acculturation into American life. Reformers often made inroads into ethnic enclaves in an attempt to Americanize newly arriving immigrants.

Jewish immigrants to the United States between 1880 and 1920 often asked themselves what it meant to be American while still retaining their Jewish identity. By the 1950s, the term "Judeo-Christian" would better express a common, melded standard and show Jewish alignment into the American body politic, and the term was even adopted by the mainstream YMCA.[37] But, in the early twentieth century, Jewish citizens were on the outside looking in.[38]

One of the major obstacles to sex education for newly arrived Jewish youth was the language difference. Margaret Sanger, opening her first birth control clinic in the Brownsville neighborhood of Brooklyn, New York, hired Russian immigrant Fania Mindell to provide translation assistance. Sanger and Mindell prepared pamphlets in English, Italian, and Yiddish to ensure that the immigrant enclaves in the area could access the information.[39] Sanger's pamphlet *What Every Girl Should Know* was also translated into Yiddish and published in 1916 and again in 1921.[40]

Ben-Zion Liber, a physician and self-proclaimed radical social reformer, took it upon himself to uplift Jewish immigrant culture in the United States through wide-ranging reforms, including sex education. He chose to write in Yiddish to address Yiddish-reading audiences, "especially . . . the kind of Jew who would read such a book in Yiddish." His publications, such as *Dos geshlekhts lebn* (Sex life) was then translated into English, reaching an even wider audience, addressing both first- and second-generation immigrants, those in the slums and those who wished to move beyond the tenement life.

Liber advocated birth control, stating that "thinking people should regulate the number of children they have" and that women could find greater meaning in life if they were able to be more than "baby machines." Like Sanger, Liber noted the demand for birth control in immigrant communities due to widespread poverty. The economic consequences of large families could be disastrous. Like Sanger and Emma Goldman, Liber used a Marxist critique of capitalism, advocating in his own way for a socialist overthrow of the current system and liberation of the people. Radical political viewpoints could limit the appeal of sex education information, or they could be useful in gaining access to labor unions and socialist societies.[41] White Christian Progressives may have seen Jewish leaders like Emma Goldman as fringe elements not only for their advocacy of public discussion about sex but because of their radical politics. Sanger, of course, distanced herself from her socialist past later in her career as she gained mainstream support. Goldman did not disavow her radical roots, and she was deported in 1917.[42]

Liber's works, including a three-hundred-page manuscript that was far more medically detailed than Sanger's books, described anatomy, pregnancy and childbirth, "normal" sexual relations, various sexual dysfunctions, and venereal diseases. More specific to Jewish audiences, it discussed the eugenic advantages of smaller families and the how sex hygiene could contribute to greater recognition of Jews as good Americans and "a credit to one's race." His newsletter, *Unzer gezund* (Our health), published letters from readers in Milwaukee, Chicago, Montreal, Denver, and even Russia. Health officials in New York also noted the reach of Liber's writing, commenting in a Health Department report in 1914 that a number of "Hebrews" mentioned *Unzer gezund* as their source for health-related information.[43]

While materials like the Yiddish translations of Sanger's pamphlets demonstrate that sex education for Jewish immigrants mirrored that available to other Americans, Liber's independent work demonstrates his interest in filling a gap in social hygiene material for the Jewish population. Sex education materials for Jewish audiences tended to also bring in the notion of building character—not for individual boys (like the YMCA) but for the Jewish community to better realize the American dream.[44]

The Boy Scouts of America

The YMCA was the principal evangelical organization for young adults at end of the nineteenth century, but by the turn of the twentieth century many reformers thought that targeting men over the age of eighteen proved less effective than going after younger boys. Progressives and physicians idealized prevention rather than cure, concluding that organizations should get to boys before they went bad. The YMCA created separate departments to work with boys under the age of eighteen, but independent groups also sought this desirable market for character building. Foremost among these groups was the Boy Scouts of America. The BSA was not specifically affiliated with a Christian denomination or evangelism, but it included a conservative moral education similar to Christian organizations.

The formation of the BSA merged two competing youth movements: the Woodcraft Indians, founded by British author and wildlife artist Ernest Thompson Seton in 1902, and the Boy Scouts founded in England by the British war hero Robert Baden-Powell. Both groups stressed character building but along very different lines. Baden-Powell emphasized militarism and preparedness while Seton's organization emphasized peace and a corrupted understanding of Native American tradition. Despite their differences, the groups laid the foundation for the American version of the Boy Scouts, which incorporated in 1910. The American BSA leadership immediately sidestepped the issue of racial segregation, concluding that scouting should be open to anyone but that local troops should determine their own memberships based on local practices. In other words, policies of separate but equal guided the early years of scouting. African Americans and Asians had to create their own troops in most areas of the country.[45]

As an alternative to authoritarian or dictatorial methods, scouting urged new methods of self-direction under the guidance of trustworthy adults. This did not mean that it was more permissive than other youth organizations. In fact, the fear of sexual precocity was prominent in its founding ideals. The Scouts aimed to channel sexual energies into other distractions: camping, exercise, and age- and sex-segregated activities.[46]

Scouting was not only supposed to provide valuable life lessons and skills to its adherents but was to occupy boys' leisure time with honest, wholesome pursuits. The first edition, published in 1913, of *The Scout Master's Handbook* described scouting as an "auxiliary to the home, school and church":

> The Scout Idea takes the non-supervised, leisure time of boys and fills it with recreation,—educational activity. . . . The preventative work of the Boy Scouts of America cannot be tabulated in statistical form but beyond question it is its largest achievement. You can sum up the whole philosophy of reaching and holding boys for all that is noble and right in one word,—pre-occupation. The fathers and mother do not fear for their boys when they are busy in school, at the factory or in the office. The time to be alarmed in their behalf is in connection with the un-accounted-for evenings . . . the time between the closing of school and supper. The Boy Scouts of America in providing helpful and character-building occupation for these hours is therefore rendering a service of inestimable importance.[47]

The BSA wished to combat juvenile delinquency (another trait of adolescence, according to Hall[48]) and sexual precocity. Boys needed supervision and a safe environment, one scouting promised to provide. Scouting was particularly popular among the middle class, who had the leisure time and resources available to dedicate to character-building pursuits.[49]

The BSA relied on scout masters to inculcate their teachings in members. *The Scout Master's Handbook* provided detailed instructions to scout masters about how to cope with the problems boys faced. The first edition required of its scout masters that they "be possessed of a *good character* because the movement in which [they work] is a moral movement and aims to build up character as well as citizenship."[50] They were to provide an example to the boys both for character and for religious faith. The BSA noted that a faithful scout master "should be a constant inspiration to the boys of his troop, causing them, no matter of how many different faiths, to be diligent in their adherence to the teachings of the particular religious institution with which they are individually connected."[51] In other words, it did not matter what a scout master believed, so long as he believed.

After outlining the requirements for masters, *The Scout Master's Handbook* sought to educate adult men about the physical and mental changes their boys would encounter during puberty, including a "shifting of ideals and a readjustment of the boy's ethical and moral viewpoint," reflecting G. Stanley Hall's theories of religious and physical storm and strife. Because of his position as adult and confidante, the scout master should "have a correct understanding and appreciation of the change as it affects the boy's life and ideals. He should be prepared to give counsel as to the care of the body, when necessary, against practices that may be dangerous to health."[52]

Scout masters had to be wary of "problem" boys, such as the sexually promiscuous or overly romantic "girl-struck boy," who developed crushes that a
scout master must channel into proper social relations, setting the stage for
later courtship. The handbook also classified nonwhite, non-middle-class boys
as potential problems but with the potential for redemption. "The Street, Foreign-Born and Negro Boys," as well as "the Wage-Earner" required additional
sympathy to overcome the difficulties of their upbringing. The manual warned
scout masters, "Some may be more shiftless than others and may need more
attention while others may be merely awaiting the touch of sympathy and the
helping hand to make strong men out of them." The manual especially urged
patience with immigrant boys, who had the potential to rise to great heights
in scouting and in society. African American boys could not as easily assim-
ilate into the white middle-class ideal, however. Thus, the manual left racial
segregation to local discretion: "economic and social conditions will naturally
determine the place of the negro boy in the Scout movement, and it is best to
leave this problem to the local councils and the Scout Masters who are directly
facing the situation."[53] Out of its own preference or out of deference to local
communities, the BSA maintained segregated troops well into the 1920s in the
North and much longer in the South.[54]

The BSA's educational program favored distraction over candid education.
Luther Gulick, who along with his wife founded the Camp Fire Girls organization, wrote in 1914, "Prevention is recognized as better and less expensive than
cure. The Boy Scout movement takes the boy at that time of life when he is
beset with the new and bewildering experiences of adolescence and diverts his
thoughts therefrom [sic] to wholesome and worth-while activities."[55] Diversion
formed a large part of the BSA's strategy regarding sexual behavior. Occasionally, the organization provided forthright information. The *Boy Scout Manual*
itself contained a legendary sex education text, one that sparked attention for
generations of scouts, in a section euphemistically entitled "Conservation":

In this chapter much has been said of the active measures which a boy should
take in order to become strong and well. We should be equally concerned
in saving and storing up natural forces we already have. In the body of every
boy, who has reached his teens, the Creator of the universe has sown a very
important fluid. This fluid is the most wonderful material in all the physical world. . . . This fluid is the sex fluid. When this fluid appears in a boy's
body, it works a wonderful change in him. His chest deepens, his shoulders
broaden, his voice changes, his ideals are changed and enlarged. It gives him
the capacity for deep feeling, for rich emotion. Pity the boy, therefore, who
has wrong ideas of this important function, because they will lower his ideals
of life. These organs actually secrete into the blood material that makes a boy
manly, strong, and noble. Any habit which a boy has that causes this fluid to
be discharged from the body tends to weaken his strength, to make him less
able to resist disease, and often unfortunately fastens upon him habits which

later in life he cannot break. Even several years before this fluid appears in the body such habits are harmful to a growing boy.

    To become strong, therefore, one must be pure in thought and clean in habit. This power which I have spoken of must be conserved, because this sex function is so deep and strong that there will come times when temptation to wrong habits will be very powerful. But remember that to yield means to sacrifice strength and power and manliness.[56]

The BSA's reticence about sex education meant that troop or scout masters did not discuss this passage with their charges. However, the presence of this passage in the manual, despite its being ignored by most BSA leaders, held immense fascination for scouts, who gathered around the campfire to puzzle over it or giggle about it. "Everyone knew the page numbers," one scout reported in the mid-twentieth century.[57]

BSA periodicals occasionally mentioned sex education. One article in *Scouting* discussed innovations among local troops. Sandwiched between a mention of fundraising efforts and the troop's mastery of the lyrics to "The Star Spangled Banner," the article stated, "One very notable feature of the work of Scout Master Irving R. Templeton . . . of Troop 15, has been the procuring of specialists to give lectures to the boys along their peculiar lines. These lectures include several along the lines of sex hygiene which have been delivered to the boys alone. It may serve as a suggestion to other Scout Masters."[58] Little evidence exists to indicate that other scout masters adopted Templeton's innovation or what was included in the lecture.

Neither the Boy Scouts nor the YMCA had created a systematic sex education program in the early twentieth century. By the early 1920s, less than one-fourth of rural YMCAs taught sex education and only six of thirty-nine local BSA units addressed the topic.[59] It seems that the Boy Scouts were more interested in distraction, while the YMCA actually tackled adolescent crises. This may have resulted from age segregation: the Scouts wished to maintain a fiction of extended boyhood, even as their older members approached adulthood. The YMCA followed through with adult education for young men and therefore may have had more of a vested interest in addressing "adult" topics.

The YMCA and the Boy Scouts could not reach all young men and boys for character development. Segregation limited their influence among African American populations in the Jim Crow South. The YMCA struggled to build black chapters because of a chronic shortage of funds to either employ secretaries or secure buildings in which to meet. Guest lecturers and reading materials cost money at a time when the South faced poverty and worsening segregation.[60] The first African American Boy Scout troops started slowly in the 1910s but likewise faced resistance from the white population as well as a chronic shortage of resources. Religiously, Catholics initially rejected the Boy

Scouts and the YMCA for their affiliation with Protestantism, although eventually Catholics accepted the BSA if led by a Catholic scout master.[61]

The practical challenges of serving a rural population were difficult, and interest in tackling such "hardened cases" was often lacking. H. Paul Douglass, writing a report of character-building organizations and their work in rural communities in 1926, complained that the YMCA, the Scouts, and similar groups failed to reach more than a handful of potential subjects. The YMCA, especially, "does not attract the most virile boys," but only the boys who would be good with or without organizational assistance.[62] Character-building groups apparently did not attract those with whom sex reformers were most concerned. The poor, immigrant, nonwhite, and isolated boys of city slums and rural backwaters neither sought nor received access to the message of sexual uplift. Reformers may have believed that these boys lacked proper sexual morality, but they either did not reach them or did not try. Small-town or suburban life was the safe middle ground. A University of Wisconsin professor accepted the conventional wisdom of urban sexual dangers but feared the perhaps even greater dangers of rural life: "County social workers have found that sex conditions in rural communities are worse from several standpoints than they are in the city. Social surveys in rural states disclose an indulgence in sex intercourse among boys and girls so widespread that it is appalling."[63] He stressed the benefits of the recent growth of organizations such as the Boy Scouts and the Camp Fire Girls, noting a "rising social feeling that play must be supervised."[64] For early twentieth-century sex educators, both the anonymity of the city and the isolation of the country led to sin. Moral rebirth thrived in small towns and suburbs where families and communities could properly supervise the sexual development of boys and girls alike. Furthermore, the YMCA and the Boy Scouts could tackle the "boy" problem to a limited extent but found themselves helpless to handle the "girl problem."

Girlhood and Sex Education

Sociologists, psychologists, and physicians saw female puberty as a completely different experience from male puberty. G. Stanley Hall's opus on adolescence was chiefly focused on males. Hall's discussion of female adolescence focused almost entirely on menstruation. His chapter entitled "Periodicity" implied that women's sexual maturation was defined chiefly by their physical struggle and less by social, emotional, or mental development.[65] There was less "storm and strife" for girls because they did not have the same opportunities as boys for education and career advancement. Girls in the early twentieth century attended high schools in greater numbers than boys, but often parents saw extended schooling not as a way to train girls for a career but as a way to prepare for and occupy time before marriage.[66] Hall noted and did not challenge many late nineteenth-century medical and educational experts who saw higher education as an unnecessary stress on adolescent girls' repro- ductive capacities.[67] Assumptions about the physical and emotional nature of girlhood resulted in a pronounced ambivalence about whether they should receive the same sort of sex education as boys should. Indeed, for several rea- sons, girls' sex education differed greatly from that aimed at boys. Boys and girls faced a different sequence of events in physical maturation. Girls often reached puberty at an earlier age than boys. The onset of menstruation, or menarche, signaled the hallmark of female puberty and was treated differ- ently from puberty in boys.

Menstruation received increased attention at the close of the nineteenth century, both for medical and hygienic reasons and for its cultural meanings.[68] As early as 1852, prominent female physician Elizabeth Blackwell worried that the age at which girls reached menarche had decreased during the nineteenth century. Specifically, she feared that wealth played a role in sexual precocity, as several studies correlated the urban upper classes with early onset of menses.[69] Common beliefs in the nineteenth century also held that working-class girls and domestic servants reached puberty and experienced regular periods before their middle-class counterparts, possibly because middle-class girls diverted energy reserved for reproductive development into education.[70] Hall's review of the pertinent literature confirmed that different groups reached menarche at different ages: he noted differences between the races, differences between residents of temperate and tropical climates, and differences between urban and rural girls.[71] Hall associated physical precocity, manifested in early men- arche, with girls outside the white middle class, even when the average age of menarche fell across the board.

Middle-class urban families encountered the drop in the age of menarche with great trepidation.[72] Victorian parents held onto an idealized age at which parents expected their daughters to enter puberty, usually around age six- teen. Since middle- and upper-class girls were in fact reaching menarche at fifteen or even fourteen by the turn of the twentieth century, even parents who intended to prepare their daughters for puberty either began instruction too late or resisted admitting that their daughters appeared by the previous gen- eration's standards to be sexually "precocious," thereby associating them with girls of other races or ethnicities. In 1897, *The Cottage Physician* put the age of menarche at fourteen and a half for girls in temperate climates, dismiss- ing "tropical" girls as precocious.[73] "Negro" and "Jewess" girls were thought to menstruate at an earlier age because of their heritage of warm climates.[74] This assumption also contributed to ideas that nonwhite girls were primitive and overly sexual. Early physical maturation was considered to be an undesirable state that imbued a class- and race-based stigma.[75]

With doctors' growing professional status, middle-class parents often turned to physicians to help guide girls through the early stages of puberty.[76] Doctors claimed that, as Joan Brumberg puts it, menstruation was "more than the punishment of Eve, and there was some actual physiology involved, physiology that medical experts could teach laypeople."[77] Learning about menstruation still remained private at the turn of the twentieth century, however. Physicians provided books or pamphlets to mothers to share with their daughters. Fournier's book for girls expressed this in its title, *For Our Daughters, When Their Mothers Judge This Advice Necessary.*[78] Winfield Scott Hall's pamphlet, *Daughter, Mother, and Father: A Story for Girls*, published by the American Medical Association in 1913, told the story of a young girl who gets advice from her physician father about anatomy but from her mother about what menstruation means for women.[79] Publications such as these stressed cooperation between the (usually male) medical expert and the (always female) trusted confidante. Menarche introduced the threat of pregnancy, therefore sparking increased interest in protecting girls from sexual predators. Physicians and mothers must face the reality of young women's developing bodies and begin gearing them toward proper courtship, marriage, and motherhood.

Medical pamphlets were eventually replaced by advice literature that accompanied commercially produced sanitary products. Historian Joan Brumberg explores how corporate marketing played a role not just in sex education but in class identities associated with the "proper" way to stay hygienic during menstruation. By the 1920s, girls viewed Kotex and other brand-name products as the height of middle-class propriety while identifying homemade rags and foreign or lower class.[80] Sex hygiene, as much as sexual behavior, had class and ethnic connotations, and the white American way of doing things was the proper way.

Contemporary assumptions about white women's low sex drive made it seem unnecessary to discourage masturbation or impure thoughts; rather, girls had to be taught to fend off the sexual advances of aggressive men.[81] One physician, Albert E. Mowry, even suggested that educating boys would alleviate the need to educate girls, since they could not get "in trouble" without boys.[82] Sex education advocate and biologist Maurice Bigelow agreed, concluding, "While an innate tendency towards general emotions of affection is strong in the average young woman, there is general absence of the localized passions that naturally and automatically develop in young men. In other words, the first definite sexual temptation is likely to come to a young woman from outside herself."[83] Therefore, sequestering girls in all-female spaces, such as girls-only schools or social organizations like the YWCA, Young Women's Hebrew Association (YWHA), the Camp Fire Girls, and the Girl Scouts, provided a suitable defense against sexual aggression.[84]

The doctrine of sexual passivity, however, had its limits. Although many authors believed that white middle-class girls lacked sex drive, either through the belief in passionlessness or because of the silence women adopted about sexuality, Bigelow did not apply the same assumptions to nonwhite or working-class girls. Bigelow took it one step farther, locating sexual purity not just in whiteness, but in American whiteness. In his sex education lectures, Bigelow included statistics of illegitimate births among women in England, France, Germany, and Sweden, to prove the superior moral character of white American girls. "It is impossible not to believe in the moral integrity of the great majority of unmarried women in America. Certainly even in our worst communities we have no such general immorality of women as . . . European figures suggest."[85] Consequently, an untimely or untoward display of sexual passion tainted girls as not fully American and not fully white. Physicians and scientists assigned different levels of sexual desire based on class, national, and race identity as well as gender.[86]

Middle-class women purity advocates saw working-class girls as a target for their efforts, assuming that they lacked a stable family environment. This same argument led to the settlement house movement in cities across America. Middle-class reformers like Jane Addams moved into a threatening neighborhood and provide services and education to those most in need. Many Progressives and settlement workers feared that working-class girls' economic instability or the desire for the trappings of middle-class material culture, be they amusements, fine clothing, or jewelry, might lead them into a life of sin. For that reason, education and protection were crucial. Margaret Cleaves, a physician writing for a Progressive journal, disagreed, arguing that all girls, "no matter what their class," needed to know the basics of anatomy and physiology. According to Cleaves, tenement life provided an opportunity for education because of its lack of privacy: "The mothers of the East Side, for example, are less apt to be negligent in the matter of necessary instruction to their daughters in connection with their sexual physiology, than mothers of better circumstances, if I may so distinguish. They are forced to this by reason of their crowded rooms and promiscuous living."[87] Cleaves saw the YWCA and working girls' clubs as a suitable alternative to schools for sex instruction.[88] City streets, especially the heterosocial dating world of dance halls, moving picture shows, and amusement parks, provided a dangerous arena for young women, especially the economically vulnerable. Women often negotiated their world with quite a bit of sexual awareness, sometimes accepting "treats" in exchange for sexual favors. Some exploitation did occur, but not all women experimented sexually under duress or in the hopes of an economic reward. Many did so to satisfy their own physical desires.[89]

Despite general assumptions about the purity of white middle-class girls, some physicians warned of a different sort of class-based danger: lesbianism. Dr. Denslow Lewis, in his controversial paper at the American Medical Association's annual conference in 1899, mentioned, "It is not my purpose, except incidentally, to refer to the perversions and unnatural practices [homosexuality] so ably described by Kraft-Ebing [*sic*]. They exist, however, in our midst, especially among young girls, to a deplorable extent, and they have their effect on women in their marital relationship." He then noted the danger of praising young girls who exhibited no interest in boys. He chided parents of the upper and middle classes who allowed their daughters to embrace, kiss, and sleep in the same bed with their female friends. "The poor, hard-working girl is not addicted to this vice. The struggle for life exhausts her capabilities. The girl brought up in luxury develops a sexual hyperesthesia [oversensitivity] which is fostered by the pleasures of modern society. She indulges in these irregular and detrimental practices, perhaps for years." Lewis did not seem overly concerned about lesbianism as a sin or a medical condition, but rather he worried that it would detract from a woman's sexual fulfillment in marriage.[90]

Fear of lesbianism illustrated both a discomfort with the Victorian tradition of romantic friendships between women and the rising awareness of homosexuality through the publications of European sexologists like Richard von Krafft-Ebing, Edward Carpenter, and Havelock Ellis. Girls who secretly read the work of sexologists occasionally recognized their own desires in the description of pathology, helping form homosexual identities later in life.[91] Same-sex environments like boarding schools provided both protection from men and temptation from women.

Other reformers expressed concerns about the perceived moral failings or hysteria of elite young women who shunned heterosexual marriage. Companionate marriage, heterosocial leisure, and the medicalization of sexuality combined to pathologize female-female relationships during the Progressive Era.[92] Physicians feared that girls who spent too much time with other girls or who had a negative or pessimistic attitude toward male sexual behavior would turn to lesbianism. Maurice Bigelow particularly wished to guide sex education advocates away from emphasizing disease and immorality, cautioning that such lessons, while effective when used with men, would scare women and prevent them from forming successful heterosexual unions. He advocated organized education as a way to counter the influence of the "extreme feministic movement" of middle-aged unmarried women who "often succeed in proselyting [sic] young women under twenty-five."[93] His advice remained class specific: "With regard to the social diseases and the social evil, I have long sympathized with the conservatives who hold that extremely limited knowledge is sufficient for the average girl under eighteen or twenty. No doubt that many working girls in cities need more protective knowledge than do school girls of the same age."[94] Reformers and educators alike associated asexuality or homosexuality with the middle and upper classes, while they reserved concern over strong heterosexual desire with the working class. In an age when eugenicists trumpeted the dangers of a lack of reproduction among the wealthiest white families, homosexuality was a threat not just to individuals or families but to the white race as well.[95] Thus, sex educators tailored their methods to reflect specific class assumptions.

For these reasons, social hygiene advocates were hesitant to "insult" the reputations of white middle class girls by advocating sex education for them. They recommended that mothers teach their daughters about menstrual hygiene so that girls did not react to menarche with fear or shock. They encouraged mothers to mention the dangers of predatory men in order to "protect" their daughters. Anything outside those two lessons was unnecessary. Therefore, sex education programs for middle-class girls were usually far more limited than those aimed at middle-class boys.

Limited—but not absent. Popular sex education author and YMCA lecturer Winfield Scott Hall aimed most of his sex education publications at boys, but he included some information about girls within those pages. In one biology-based hygiene text, he included a brief discussion of a girl's entry into woman-hood. He advised girls to rest and avoid vigorous activities during "expulsion of the ovum," although he makes no mention of menstruation.[96] A few years later, Hall published a work aimed at girls, entitled *Daughter, Mother, and Father: A Story for Girls.* Because of the change in audience, as well as the six-year difference between his early work and this one, Hall gave a more complete picture of menstruation. He still advised decreased physical activity, but he noted that menstruation is normal, not pathological.[97]

By the 1910s, Winfield Scott Hall found himself in competition with a new crop of female physicians and reformers who wished to demystify puberty for girls. Before she gained worldwide fame through her advocacy of birth control, Margaret Sanger began her public career as a nurse and socialist activist in New York's Greenwich Village. Sanger's firsthand experience as a public nurse in New York's poorest neighborhoods helped lead to her activism for better distri-bution of knowledge and, later, contraception, for the women there. In 1911, she published sex education articles in the New York *Call*, a socialist newspaper. Her first series of articles, "What Every Mother Should Know," discussed how to educate one's children on the facts of life. Sanger's first series was steeped in Victorian niceties (perhaps in an attempt to avoid prosecution), describing ways in which mothers could teach their children the "facts of life," beginning with plant life and moving up to more complex life forms. Sanger's first articles rarely confronted Victorian ideas about human sexuality in between her tales of "Mr. and Mrs. Buttercup" and "Mr. and Mrs. Frog." In fact, she reinforced the Victorian cultural construct of mothers as the guardians of moral, reli-gious, and cultural values to be passed on to the children.[98] The only change lay in Sanger's medium: the newspaper instead of the home.[99]

The next year, Sanger's second series, "What Every Girl Should Know," changed the target audience from parents to the girls themselves and expanded the lessons given. Her work democratized knowledge, insisting that women's education and raised consciousness were vital steps toward political and economic revolution. Throughout the second series, Sanger stressed the duty to provide accurate information to those who needed it. Particularly, she believed that the working classes required better education than they received, but she did not stress working-class girls' sexual vulnerability or desire. Rather,

Sanger argued that working girls were the group most likely to lack another reliable source of medical and sexual information. Middle- and upper-class women could have their questions answered by private physicians; poor women, unable to afford private doctors, suffered most from the unevenly implemented Comstock Laws.[100]

Challenging the emerging notion of Progressive physicians that menstruation did not adversely affect a girl's energy, Sanger wrote, "The average girl in this country spends two days of pain and discomfort." Her prolabor sympathies aroused, Sanger argued, "To the girl who has to work from early morning until late at night, these two days are unusually hard on her nerves and on her general health, and I regret that I have no new message for her to help lighten the burden, which under the present atrocious industrial system makes it so hard for her." She concluded that, accordingly, a girl should insist on "at least one day's rest at the expense of her employer. . . . It is a time women should band together in one great sisterhood to protect one another from being slowly drained and exhausted of their powers of motherhood for the benefit of their exploiters."[101] Thus, menstruation became a reason for female solidarity in the workplace and another reason to condemn industrial capitalism. She stated that wealthy girls attending the finer schools received special consideration during menses, "and it is well that this is so." Sanger thought that the class divide between working girls and schoolgirls showed once again the inhumanity of the capitalist system as a threat to girls' health and the future of the race.[102]

Sanger provided very forthright advice for avoiding pregnancy in her popular pamphlet *Family Limitation*, first published in 1914. In it, she provided information on conception, douching, condoms, and pessaries (diaphragms), advising women to take charge of their own health care to prevent unwanted pregnancies. Sanger used scientifically correct terminology, not shying away from words like "penis" and "vagina" and presented practical advice without the overlay of moral and spiritual proselytizing. Her pragmatic approach included a detailed lesson on female anatomy, arguing that if women were to use the pessary (her preferred method of contraception), they must be knowledgeable about their own anatomy: "the trouble is women are afraid of their own bodies, and are of course ignorant of their physical construction." Her pamphlet was quite popular, going through six printings in the first three years.[103] Sanger explicitly linked women's rights to women's knowledge of (and control over) their bodies in *Family Limitation* as well as her newsletters, *The Woman Rebel* and the *Birth Control Review*. Sanger wrote in her first issue of *The Woman Rebel* in 1914, "It is hoped the young girl will derive some knowledge of her nature, and conduct her life upon such knowledge." Sanger promised to use her platform to teach girls and women about contraception, sexual hygiene, and "at all times the WOMAN REBEL will advocate women's economic emancipation." There was as much labor activism in her early publications as sex education or birth control.[104]

Like Sanger, physician Clelia Duel Mosher agreed that women's health was crucial to a revolution in women's rights. Mosher worked at Stanford University as a hygiene instructor and the campus women's medical advisor. In 1915, Mosher addressed an audience at the Fourth Biennial Conference of the YWCA on the topic of female health reform, arguing that society's *assumptions* about menstruation, and not menstruation itself, was the reason women got sick. Mosher echoed Sanger's plea for more expansive sex education, but Mosher believed education would solve the supposed pathology: "if every young girl were taught that menstruation is not normally a 'bad time' and that pain or incapacity at that period is as discreditable and unnecessary as bad breath due to decaying teeth, we might almost look for a revolution in the physical life of women."[105] Mosher's use of the word "revolution" was not an exaggeration. She saw concrete connections between the way male physicians interpreted women's health concerns and the overall oppression of women in patriarchal American society. Health and sexual education were cornerstones to women realizing full equality with men. Therefore, the work of physicians, educators, and community organizations such as the YWCA were all the more important: "a great responsibility rests upon us as physicians and teachers of physical training to lead women to ideas of health."[106]

Character-building organizations did not promote the revolution in knowledge Mosher or Sanger suggested. Many middle-class reformers perceived women like Sanger as dangerous radicals with anarchist and socialist connections. Instead, they continued the trend of assuming that sex education for girls centered on protecting purity. One character-building organization, the YWCA, trained a lecturer on sex hygiene for a tour in 1914, noting that the organization felt "under obligation to promote knowledge of the fundamental facts of life, to arouse a sympathetic attitude toward them, and to call forth the power whereby this knowledge shall make for individual and community morality." The YWCA hired Dr. Mabel Ulrich of Minneapolis, Minnesota, to present talks in high school biology classes and at YWCA meetings.[107] The YWCA provided a more limited program than the YMCA, including some hygiene and character training to young women in their purview.

The YWCA grew extensively during the 1910s, although it remained a largely white, Protestant, and northern phenomenon. By 1919, 360 associations had been organized throughout the nation, expanding their work with young women. Following the lead of its male counterpart, the YWCA maintained racial segregation in keeping with local tradition and as a way to woo white southern women into the organization. While they allowed black women's chapters, white women regularly assumed they would maintain control over black chapters.[108] The YWCA also recognized that different audiences required different work, and so they organized programs in "religious education, work for girls from Foreign-speaking homes, Colored Work, [and] Open Country [rural areas]."[109]

The organization typically used coded language to address concerns about the moral and sexual purity of both its volunteers and its members. In *A Handbook for Leaders of Younger Girls*, the YWCA advised, "Between the ages of twelve and eighteen, every girl goes through certain psychological as well as physiological changes. An understanding of these changes helps a club leader immeasurably." It also advised leaders to exhibit "self-control," both for their own good and to provide a model to their charges. The most forthright segment of social hygiene training was in the section on athletics. The handbook notes:

> Girls of adolescent age are not apt to be greatly interested in regular lectures on health. Certain fundamental facts which all girls should possess can be given by any well-informed woman in five- or ten-minute rest periods which come during the athletic work. The girls' attention is then directed toward her body and she is interested in knowing the ways by which she can make and keep it as beautiful as possible. Much valuable information can be given in such ten-minute talks during the year.[110]

The emphasis on beauty, which places both girls' athletic "work" and their health concerns into the frame of physical attractiveness, discounts the more empowering messages of Mosher, Sanger, and even YWCA lecturer Mabel Ulrich. The YWCA handbook seemed to assume that women required no special medical training and that a full-fledged hygiene lecture was unnecessary and uninteresting to most girls.[111]

Groups like the YWCA and the Girls Scouts tended to be as timid and euphemistic as the groups for men and boys. Juliette Gordon Low, a well-traveled widow and acquaintance of Robert Baden-Powell, founded the Girl Scouts in Savannah, Georgia, in 1912, borrowing liberally from Baden-Powell's English program, the Girl Guides. She adopted similar uniforms, organizational names, and portions of their handbook. Patterned after the BSA, the Girl Scouts was an organization designed to guide preadolescent and adolescent girls through educational, physical, and spiritual development. Low wished to bring girls out of the isolation of the home and into community service.[112] The Girl Scouts also segregated troops based on race, with the first African American troop formed in 1917. The Girl Scouts created segregated troops for blacks, Mexican Americans, and American Indians in accordance with local segregation laws and customs.[113]

The 1920 edition of the *Girl Scout Manual* emphasized the importance of keeping clean and hygienic. Unlike the *Boy Scout Manual*, however, the word "sex" was not included:

> Every Girl Scout knows the deep and vital need for clean and healthy bodies in the mothers of the next generation. This not only means keeping her skin fresh and sweet and her system free from every impurity, but it goes far

deeper than this, and requires every Girl Scout to respect her body and mind so much that she forces everyone else to respect them and keep them free from the slightest familiarity or doubtful stain.[114]

The language was coded, but the message of purity as a requirement to the success of eventual motherhood came through. Even this message was quite an expansion from the first Girl Scout book, the 1913 edition of *How Girls Can Help Their Country*. This precursor to the *Girl Scout Manual* updated the standard Boy Scout Law to cultivate "honor, duty, loyalty, kindness, comradeship, purity, cheerfulness, and thrift" among scouts. Purity replaced cleanliness in the girls' version. The only other implicit reference to menstruation is the instruction that "no girl must bathe when not well." Perhaps the 1913 edition was even more tentative because it was written by a man, W. J. Hoxie. Whatever the reason, the author specifically aimed the book at adult scouting leaders, thus interposing another level of censorship on topics of interest to the girls themselves.[115]

The Girl Scouts did not provide the only image of idealized girlhood during the Progressive Era. Luther Gulick, a physician and social activist, founded the Camp Fire Girls in 1910 with his wife, Charlotte. Their goal was not to create a female version of the newly established Boy Scouts but to create a complementary group that would utilize some of the same concepts of outdoor life and character development, while at the same time embracing distinctions between masculinity and femininity. The Camp Fire Girls used the symbol of the domestic fire or hearth to center their energies on women's roles as mothers, caregivers, and helpmates.[116] Yet the ideology of domesticity and femininity was combined with outdoor activities and camaraderie to develop a more complete and healthy young woman. The Camp Fire organization, nonsectarian and interracial in keeping with the beliefs of its founders, was significantly more popular than the Girl Scouts until after the 1920s. Yet it was still dominated by middle-class white Christians.[117]

Like the Girl Scouts, the Camp Fire Girls officially endorsed purity in the realm of sex education. In discussing the importance of Indian ritual, Charles A. Eastman, the Native American writer and reformer, claimed to adapt an Indian ceremony suitable for Camp Fire Girls. In the ceremony, the girls were encouraged to take the "maiden's vow":

> Upon this stone I take the maiden's twofold vow;
> the vow of purity—my duty to myself;
> the pledge of service—my duty to others.[118]

Owing to the contested understanding of girls' adolescence, sexual interest, and the meaning of puberty, few character-building organizations designed for girls were willing to call attention to anything other than purity or the barest lessons in bodily hygiene. Sex education for girls remained largely a question of protecting "innocent" girls from sexual predators. Mothers remained the appropriate instructor.

Character-building organizations rooted their reform efforts in specific ideas about gender, race, and class. Created by white middle-class reformers and largely segregated by race and sex, they often did not adequately reach, or allow significant voices of, youth outside the white middle class. Racially segregated organizations lagged behind in access and resources, and they often had to cope with paternalistic, racist, or dismissive national administrators. The working definition of adolescence as a time of storm and strife, of sexual awakening and the inherent dangers that came with it, demanded a response from male-focused groups like the YMCA and the BSA. They taught the importance of chivalry, Christian manhood, a single sexual standard, and boys' duties as the leaders and parents of tomorrow. Prior to World War I, disease prevention, anatomy, and physiology seemed less vital than social purity lessons: respect for women, racial purity, and an effort to prolong childhood and distract boys from their burgeoning sexual feelings.[119] A pioneer in the field, the YMCA attempted to provide age-appropriate hygiene education in addition to moral admonitions to stay pure. The Boy Scouts resisted taking on the burden of sex education, leaving the topic largely out of their realm. Both groups urged healthy preoccupations for growing boys—outdoor exercise, nature study, sports, and skill development—in an effort to reduce sexual precocity and save the middle-class white boy from the dangers of the modern, urban world.

When the topic shifted to girls, resistance to sex education increased. Some radical feminists linked health information to political equality, but organizational efforts to provide sex education to girls remained limited by the stereotype of "passionless" middle-class girlhood. Only a few radical voices like Margaret Sanger and Emma Goldman pushed the envelope—and ran afoul of the law for their efforts. Mainstream organizations like the YWCA and the Girl Scouts avoided the topic. Even condemning the lack of sex education could be interpreted as somehow sullying white middle-class girls' reputations. Consequently, sex education for girls lagged behind efforts for their male counterparts.

Built on assumptions of social privilege and a framework of Christian purity, character-building organizations constructed class, gender, and racial identity as much as morality or ethics. Consequently, middle-class white boys received sex education, but a version that separated their experience of sexual maturation from that of others. African Americans and others who did not fit the mold—the "problem boys" of the *Scout Master's Handbook*—had to seek alternative paths.

Chapter Four

Venereal Disease and Sex Education for African Americans

In December 1914, Dr. Barnett M. Rhetta of Baltimore, Maryland, read a paper before the Maryland Medical, Dental, and Pharmaceutical Association. Rhetta was a well-known black physician in the area, a leading member of the National Medical Association and an advocate for black representation in public health associations. His paper, entitled "A Plea for the Lives of the Unborn," raised some sticky subjects, especially for black physicians in the early twentieth century. Rhetta argued that physicians must not help people have fewer children but instead must advocate on behalf of the unborn. Rhetta furiously denied the legitimacy of contraception and abortion, recognizing a large problem in the debate over reproductive health for African Americans: eugenics. Rhetta declared, "Eugenics has been defined as 'That science which deals with influences that improve the unborn qualities of the race.' In other words, it is that science which tends to improve mankind by breeding better children." Rhetta noted the purported benefit of this idea: "When properly applied, there is no higher calling in the field of medicine. But to you, and for me, as practiced here today, it means death." He continued, "Cranks . . . have spread it that in the name of Eugenics and for the betterment of the race, the Negro in America should be silently wiped out."[1] Here was the crux of Rhetta's quandary. How could he support greater access to contraception or abortion without playing into the hands of white supremacists who wished to eliminate the black race?

Rhetta's fervent rejection of contraception reflected the very ambiguous relationship between race and contraception. Black and white doctors, each claiming medical expertise, applied the politics of racial betterment (or racial survival) to their own political aims. Whereas white supremacists expressed the wish to see African Americans quarantined from infecting the sexual health of whites, black doctors challenged scientific racism and saw the debate over sexual hygiene and birth control through their own lens of racial solidarity, survival, and respectability.

Interestingly, Rhetta reappears in the press a few decades later. In 1955, *Jet Magazine* noted that Dr. Barnett M. Rhetta, age seventy-one, was found guilty of performing illegal abortions, though he was given probation "because of his age and health and his past good record."[2] Abortion was a family business, as police arrested Rhetta's son and namesake both in 1955 and 1967 for performing illegal abortions.[3] What prompted Rhetta to so completely change his mind regarding reproductive rights that he would break the law to provide women an option to not have children? Dr. Rhetta's ideas on racial betterment and respectability influenced his evolving stance on reproductive rights.

The early social hygiene movement, exemplified by the American Social Hygiene Association's formation in 1914 under racist eugenicist Charles Eliot, did not mince words: it focused on preserving the moral and physical integrity of the white population in the United States. Its emphasis on character building, especially among middle-class boys and men, further marginalized people outside the white community. Sex education for African American youths, in particular, was not a high priority among white reformers. Indeed, many social hygiene reformers saw sex education for racial minorities as futile.

Progressive whites, especially but not exclusively in the South, reduced sex education for African Americans to a rudimentary form of syphilis prevention or quarantine. They believed that blacks were a "syphilis-soaked race"[4] lacking in morals and that the sort of education Progressives advocated for whites, stressing chivalry and moral suasion, would prove useless. Instead, their efforts relied on preventing syphilis from spreading beyond the black community. This philosophy demonstrates the underlying goals of social control and self-preservation among white Progressives who ostensibly espoused education and uplift to better society. It also highlights how racial separation played a major role in the white Progressive crusade in the South.[5] The sex education movement complemented broader Progressive-Era racial restrictions: Jim Crow segregation, decreased black political power, and denial of public health care and education to African Americans. Ideologies of racial purity connected the sex education movement and the popular eugenics movement in the name of science.

This chapter traces the medical and social debates surrounding sex education for African Americans in the prewar South. Building on stereotypes supported by scientific racism, white medical professionals blamed blacks for high rates of venereal disease and dismissed as hopeless efforts to treat the disease. Unwilling to accept such dismissals, black medical professionals created their own sex education curricula, often countering racist arguments about black immorality with a class-based argument of racial uplift. They utilized the language of racial duty, clearly delineated gender roles, and the centrality of the black church to fight sexual immorality and to prove their respectability. Despite fears of whites using eugenic arguments against blacks, many black elites even championed elements of eugenic arguments to improve "the race" by increasing the number of African American elites. Black elites hoped to separate themselves from both the dominant stereotypes of the white community and what they considered the real problem of the poor majority.[6] Class, as well as race and gender, shaped the strategies, tactics, and goals of medical professionals and sex education reformers on both sides of the color line.[7]

Black Adolescence

Just as G. Stanley Hall analyzed white adolescence, scientists and researchers examined racial differences in the development of young people across the races. In the late nineteenth century, the rise in status of the physician, along with the rise in visibility of the social sciences like sociology and anthropology, led to a greater curiosity about what made humans different or the same. Most proponents of rigid racial hierarchies believed that biology, anthropology, religion, and sociology scientifically and dispassionately explained the roots of racial difference.

By the height of US colonial empire building in the late nineteenth century, theories of anatomical difference predominated, placing Africans below Europeans when whites ranked the peoples of the world, owing not to their culture but to their faulty bodies.[8] White colonialists argued that Africans stayed mentally childlike forever, thus justifying white stewardship over them.[9] Europeans justified colonial expansion into other nations in part through a belief in recapitulation, arguing that each society or race traveled along the same path toward civilization, with the white race clearly furthest along the path.[10] Race and recapitulation were concepts that combined anthropology and biology, cultural ideas and apparent physical differences.[11]

In the eyes of white supremacists, blacks were concomitantly the "innocent primitive" and the "uncontrollable primitive"—perpetual children and perpetual sexual beings. This flouted the early twentieth-century construction of white adolescence as a period of sexual awakening and internal struggle toward maturity.[12] Since reformers labeled adolescence as the time when sex education was supposed to protect the moral and physical development of children, sex education for African Americans seemed useless if they did not experience a comparable period of adolescence.

Sexuality became a way of marking racial and class differences. White reformers saw sexual repression as part of their identity and a reason for their ability to wield power over other races. In some settings nonwhites adopted the sexual standards of the white middle class in an attempt to elevate their own class and racial status.[13] American medical attitudes focused on race as a key factor in physical, biological, and emotional development. White physicians and sociologists used race as the determining factor contributing to black children's development and, as a result, developed a theory of black adolescence starkly opposed to G. Stanley Hall's. By framing race as a biological phenomenon, scientists (falsely) claimed greater objectivity than social theorists.

Experts attempted to demonstrate this objectivity by noting the purported advantages blacks possessed. The 1910 edition of the famed *Encyclopedia Britannica* included the following in its entry on the Negro by British Museum archaeologist Thomas Athol Joyce:

> The remark of F[ilippo] Manetta, made after a long study of the negro in America, may be taken as generally true of the whole race: "the negro children were sharp, intelligent and full of vivacity, but on approaching the adult period a gradual change set in. The intellect seemed to become clouded, animation giving place to a sort of lethargy, briskness yielding to indolence. We must necessarily suppose that the development of the negro and white proceed on different lines."[14]

Black children could excel only until they reached puberty. Joyce attributed different paths of physical development to the supposed anatomical differences between whites and blacks. Joyce assumed blacks had an all-encompassing interest in sexuality:

> While with the [white] the volume of the brain grows with the expansion of the brainpan, in the [negro] the growth of the brain is on the contrary arrested by the premature closing of the cranial sutures and lateral pressure on the frontal bone. This explanation is reasonable and even probable as a contributing cause; but evidence is lacking on the subject and the arrest or even deterioration in mental development is no doubt very largely due to the fact that after puberty sexual matters take the first place in the negro's life and thoughts.[15]

By assigning the cause of racial differences to anatomical differences, scientists gave credence to denigrating stereotypes and pushed blacks into a category as "other." They linked physical development to sexual expression, once again attributing what they termed immoral behavior to blacks' "natural" progression through a stunted puberty. The rising professional status of physicians at this time gave weight to such judgments. Reliance on sociological evidence of community behavior could seem contentious, whereas "hard" scientific or medical evidence was thought to be above debate. Assigning causation to scientific evidence was less likely to be called into question in the early twentieth century, when a regulated and educated profession came to prominence in the United States.[16]

Anatomical determinism did not stay confined to medical circles. In his 1910 treatise on racial development, white sociologist Howard Odum wrote, "Negro children are easily interested, attentive, eager, and alert. For the most part, they are bright and learn easily." But the praise quickly faded. "As a rule, after Negro children become older than ten or twelve years, their development is physical rather than mental; whatever of mental ability in the child gave promise of worth to be recognized in later years is crowded out by the coarser physical growth."[17] Their bodies, he argued, continued to grow while their minds stagnated at puberty. As a result, black children grew into uncontrolled sexual beings with childish minds. Odum wrote that blacks were "lacking in morals, so far as personal purity and chastity are concerned."[18] This fed into a widespread white belief that blacks were promiscuous, and particularly that black men wanted to sexually assault white women. Odum's sociological and biological argument supported whites' fears of black male rapists.[19]

The white-dominated American medical profession put forth a purportedly scientific understanding of black adolescence and sexual development, assuming that the "normal" black was not the same as the "normal" white. Building on such a foundation of racialized medicine, adding shoddy statistics and anecdotal evidence, white doctors stressed the enfeebled nature of blacks both in Africa and in the American South. Chief among their concerns was syphilis.

The Venereal Peril—Scourge of the Race?

Army physician Dr. Edward Bright Vedder published his monograph, *Syphilis and Public Health*, in 1918, at the height of the venereal scare in the United States. Vedder, who had served in the Philippines and was considered an expert on tropical medicine, did not allow the Great War to distract him from his focus on the distinction of race. He wrote, "Whites and negroes should, of course, be considered separately" when studying venereal diseases.[20] His work included gender as well as racial stereotypes, noting that white women and people of color were both anatomically inferior to white men. Particularly, he indicted women of African descent as the scourge of white society. Echoing colonial medical theories, he accused black women of increasing VD rates tenfold in Africa: "The reason is that the women, whether married or single, practically all have intercourse with the whites" who colonized Africa. Their promiscuity, a factor of race and gender, also damned women, since he theorized that immoral women had many more sexual partners than immoral men.[21] He then applied his theory to African Americans: "this fact explains the higher incidence of syphilis among the negro women in the United States."[22] Vedder's reliance on racial and gendered thought shaped the entire body of his work on venereal disease and indeed his analysis of American civilization as a whole, as demonstrated by his aphorism, "It is probable that whole races become thoroughly syphilized much faster than they become civilized."[23] VD was both a biological event and a socially constructed reflection of cultural values and beliefs.[24]

Did African Americans, as Vedder claimed, have higher rates of syphilis and other sexually transmitted diseases in the early twentieth century than their white counterparts? Most contemporary writers admitted that no reliable statistics existed in the late nineteenth or early twentieth century to prove that allegation. Public health was in its infancy. Many who suffered from venereal diseases turned to irregular treatments or home remedies to find a cure, and VD was not required to be reported as were other contagious diseases. But that did not prevent an outpouring of self-proclaimed experts who put forth their own numbers. A review of medical literature from the early twentieth century attributed the rates of venereal infection among blacks to be anywhere from 5 to 90 percent! Indeed, many physicians denied the necessity of numbers to tell readers what they intuitively "knew": blacks were nearly universally infected with VD.[25]

Prior to World War I, many in the medical press remained reticent about sexual health in general, making the rare mention of VD noteworthy. An article published in the journal *Medicine* in 1903 combined the same sorts of anthropological and medical rhetoric that Vedder used to disparage black sexuality. In addition to a half-dozen popular sex education books, the Connecticut white physician and world traveler William Lee Howard published "The Negro as a Distinct Ethnic Factor in Civilization," an article that contained little medical or scientific information. Howard attacked white northern philanthropists for ignoring the biological reasons for racial segregation. He denigrated education, charity work, and integration as dangerous actions that would not reduce the fundamental differences between the races: "the belief that the African was capable of living as hygienically and morally as the Caucasian was the great mistake made by those who deal in abstract principles." Physicians, he added, know the false nature of these abstracts, because they have to cope with the concrete problems of insanity, tuberculosis, and syphilis. His solution: strict segregation. "There is every prospect of checking and reducing these diseases in the white race, if this race is socially—in every aspect of the term—quarantined from the African." Howard developed a strong believed in the benefits of sex education for whites, authoring numerous books designed for (white) boys and girls in the 1910s. Yet according to his 1903 article, no amount of treatment, training, preventive work, or education could solve the problem of sexual hygiene for the black population. Therefore, the only logical solution was to save the white race from any interaction with blacks.[26]

White physicians across the South echoed Howard's support of strict segregation to contain VD. In 1906, the *American Journal of Dermatology and Genito-Urinary Diseases* published two articles by white southern physicians echoing Howard's viewpoint. Georgia physician Henry McHatton published "The Sexual Status of the Negro—Past and Present," only gesturing toward an attempt to bring more hard science into the discussion. He began by stating, "There are no statistics available for an article of this description. One has to depend on personal observation and the opinion of others who are in a position to have experience along these lines."[27] But his experience living on a slave plantation in the "old regime" American South and in pre-emancipation Cuba, as well as his medical practice in Georgia, made him a self-appointed authority. He concluded that slavery had provided a salubrious state for African Americans; as valuable property, it was in the owners' best interest to maintain their health and happiness. McHatton unhesitatingly stated, "No race of human beings ever lived as healthy a life as the plantation negro in the South and in Cuba."[28]

McHatton used venereal disease as evidence of the decay of African American health after emancipation. He argued that after 1865, the freedmen paid "no attention to the most elementary laws of hygiene."[29] He placed the blame squarely on the shoulders of nature rather than social or economic circumstances: "they are naturally nomads, and are on the go all the time." Mobility, he argued, contributed to a culture of widespread prostitution, unstable marriages, and near-universal levels of venereal infection. Connecting his ideas to recapitulation theory, McHatton added, "His rapid degeneration, physically, mentally and morally, and his reversion to barbaric tendencies, with all the added vices of civilization, is appalling. From the most healthy race in the country, forty years ago, he is today the most diseased."[30]

Another white Georgia physician, Dr. Daniel David Quillian, agreed that African heritage physically doomed African Americans. In "Racial Peculiarities: A Cause of the Prevalence of Syphilis in Negroes," Quillian noted the lack of reliable statistics, but since he was a white southern doctor, he claimed the expertise necessary to explain the problem: "The negro, by virtue of the fact that he is a native naturally of tropical and semitropical climates, has his sexual instincts developed to a very high degree. . . . By virtue of this inordinate desire for sexual gratification, and because of their lax morals and indifference to virtue, the negro as a race is more prone to venereal disease than the white race."[31] He then estimated that 60–70 percent of blacks in the South had either hereditary or acquired syphilis. This was higher than McHatton's conservative estimate of at least 25 percent in the active stages of syphilis, although McHatton pointed out that he did not attempt to calculate the percentage suffering from gonorrhea or syphilis in the inactive stage.[32] Quillian admitted that those numbers might shock his readers, but he insisted that they were accurate and acceptable if one understood "the fact that the negro has a peculiar tolerance for the disease" and thus it was often undiagnosed and went without treatment. Unsure where this "partial immunity" originated, Quillian theorized that it might be due to active outdoor work or a hereditary benefit of being a "blighted race" for so many generations.[33]

Both writers revealed one of their biggest concerns about African American health: reproduction.[34] Lacking reliable statistics, Quillian and McHatton noted that, in their personal experience, the birth rate among African Americans had dropped significantly after emancipation. Both attributed the plunge in black birth rates to high rates of venereal disease, which can cause sterility.[35] Modern scholarship has challenged their assertion, attributing at least part of the fertility rate drop to black women's improved access to contraception such as douches. Many black women embraced birth control as a way to ease economic pressures and exert control over their lives and their families, a power previously denied to enslaved women.[36] Apparently, it did not occur to McHatton and Quillian that black women might have consciously planned their pregnancies. Rather, these two physicians assumed that their own observations and conclusions, interpreted solely from their personal experience, represented black southerners as a whole.

Besides fertility rates, whites and blacks alike discussed the troubling issue of infant mortality among the black population. While statistics remained elusive, both blacks and whites concurred that infant mortality rates were particularly high among African Americans. However, what white "experts" deemed a sign of racial degeneracy, blacks interpreted to be a result of poverty and lack of quality medical care.[37] High infant mortality rates may have made black women cautious about undergoing repeated pregnancies and thus more interested in contraception. Even against a background of eugenics and talk of racial destiny, women still desired individual control over fertility. And if women were willing to challenge the strictures of their own community, they certainly distrusted racist rhetoric from white professionals.[38]

White southern physicians steeped their assumptions about black health in paternalism. Reminiscent of the debates over emancipation and Reconstruction, white southerners resisted northern interference with their own "peculiar" style of race relations. They wanted to control the scientific debate and control the methods of solving what they conceptualized as a problem. Framing it as southern whites' duty to protect the health of blacks showcased how whites supposedly cared about blacks, and how they were the ones who could best solve blacks' problems. Indeed, southern physicians often used their status as southerners to dismiss the possibility of race prejudice, assuring readers that they could not be prejudiced against a group that they encountered with such intimacy in daily life. One book review in the *Southern Medical Journal* noted that southern practitioners "are close students of the Negro problem, and . . . are best informed regarding the physical deterioration of the American negro that is manifest to every unprejudiced observer."[39] Another physician prefaced an article on preventive health care for blacks by writing, "Being a Southern man by birth and preference, nothing said in this article can be construed as an attack upon the Negro."[40] Another assured, "No other people in the world knows [the Negro] as we do, likes him as we do, tolerates him as we do."[41] The South was certainly not the only region where racial prejudice existed in medicine. Assumptions about the medical and social failings of African Americans permeated the entire country, but southern physicians and their local and regional medical associations argued that they ought to lead the discussion, owing to their proximity to the largely southern black population.

Southern medical journals encouraged paternalistic medical practice, but even the most eminent national medical publication did not shy away from similar themes. For instance, the *Journal of the American Medical Association* (*JAMA*) also printed southern physicians' spurious arguments in the name of science. In March of 1910, *JAMA* published a lengthy article entitled "Syphilis and the American Negro: A Medico-Sociological Study." Virginia doctor Thomas Murrell claimed for himself not just the expertise of his profession but also expertise based on his identity as a white southerner just as Quillian and McHatton had. He argued that while reliable statistics on disease among blacks in the South were lacking, he offered several "well-known facts" in his article. "Morality among these people is almost a joke and only assumed as a matter of convenience . . . and venereal disease is well-nigh universal. As an illustration of this: In clinic and private practice I have never seen a negro virgin over 18 years of age."[42] Whether they attributed black women's purported lack of morality to postemancipation social chaos, tropical blood, or an anthropological attraction to immorality, many southern white physicians concurred that African American women were immoral.[43] Even more, all African Americans were doomed to a short-lived future of venereal disease, infertility, and death. Rather than public health, prophylaxis, or education, the white medical community posited that the solution to the VD problem was to keep it out of the white community by strict racial segregation, while letting the problem solve itself through high mortality and declining birth rates among blacks. Adopting eugenic language and social Darwinism, many in the white medical establishment assumed blacks would die out naturally.

Black Professionals Respond

White physicians, sociologists, anthropologists, and reformers debated the sources of black pathology while newly emerging black professionals publicly questioned the very foundation of their arguments. Dr. John A. Kenney, school physician and hospital director at Tuskegee University, challenged medical journals that made racial attacks under the guise of scientific objectivity. In 1909, Kenney wrote, "When men high in the medical profession use the leading medical journals of the country to assail and libel a whole race of people, it is time that our one publication should speak and speak plainly."[44] Kenney endeavored to refute Thomas Murrell's "well-known facts." The lack of statistics made it as hard to negate as to prove such arguments, and blacks fought an uphill battle against persistent racial stereotypes.

One of the major problems black physicians had in confronting accusations of disease was that they lacked the same sort of professional respect and recognition that formal organizations such as the AMA granted white physicians. A group of African American medical professionals founded the National

Medical Association in 1895 to counter the exclusionary practices practiced and tolerated by the AMA. The AMA, the largest and most influential medical organization in the United States, used a federated membership system. It allowed its local chapters to determine who could gain local membership, which then formed their national membership. Consequently, state and county associations, particularly in the South, could restrict their memberships to whites only. This policy effectively prevented African American physicians from having a voice in this powerful political and scientific organization.[45]

The NMA set out to develop medical schools, hospitals, and residency training programs to counter the AMA's segregation. Its motto, as ascribed in the 1909 *Journal of the National Medical Association* (*JNMA*), stated that the NMA was "conceived in no spirit of racial exclusiveness, fostering no ethnic antagonism, but born of the exigencies of American environment, the National Medical Association has for its object the banding together for mutual co-operation and helpfulness."[46] The NMA, formed in response to professional segregation, took as its larger aim an effort to end racial discrepancies in health, especially mortality and morbidity rates, and to expand access to health-care services for needy African Americans.

Central to this goal, the NMA leadership attempted to bolster the reputations of black health professionals, both among African Americans in the South and among blacks and whites in the nation as a whole. Professionalization, they believed, would accomplish two things. First, they wished to place black middle-class health-care professionals at the forefront of their communities in order to lead them in health reform. Second, they wished to demonstrate to the white community that blacks could master the sciences and counter the racist arguments the white medical establishment had adopted. More than anything, the NMA wished to correct what they considered the dual causes of high black mortality and morbidity: lack of knowledge and lack of access to health care (both related to segregation and poverty). Kenney argued that high rates of black mortality from diseases such as tuberculosis were due not to some sort of anatomical fault but "to acquired conditions partly forced upon the race from the exterior and partly from his own personal neglect and ignorance."[47] This statement demonstrated that black professionals tended to reproach the less educated, attributing to working-class African Americans some of the same stereotypes that whites applied to the black race as a whole.

The black medical elite focused on improving race relations as well as hygiene and morality in order to improve the health of the masses. The *JNMA* extemporized on morals as much as on science. This was not uncommon in early twentieth-century medical journals. *JAMA* and lesser mainstream medical journals commonly included both editorials and articles that discussed moral judgments as much as health issues. Like their white counterparts, black medical professionals sought to shore up their influence and establish their role as moral and intellectual leaders. Kenney discussed how the NMA planned to work in conjunction with other middle-class and aspirational organizations: "go forth and take an active part in the fight and preach the 'Gospel of Good Health and Right Living.'"[48] Overtly linking religion and morality to health, Kenney and other prominent *JNMA* contributors considered it their duty to lift up their less-informed brethren and to present a good image to the white mainstream.

The NMA was part of a larger effort on the part of the black middle class—and those aspiring to middle-class status—to uplift the race, seen in organizations like the National Association of Colored Women. Black clubwomen adopted the motto "lifting as we climb" to denote their efforts to help those around them as well as improve their own lives.[49] Duty to the race took form in the physician's role to educate and heal the masses, the mother's role to raise the next generation, and the role of the wealthy to assist the poor.[50] Racial uplift served to help the poor as well as to provide the middle class with a sense of class identity and purpose. They did not advocate or expect a classless society.

Many black professionals and aspiring professionals thought class distinctions among blacks were healthy. Charles V. Roman, editor of the *JNMA*, wrote in his book, *American Civilization and the Negro* (1916), "The persistent effort to treat all colored people alike retards the healthful growth of class distinction among us and lessens the influence of the intelligent and virtuous over the ignorant and vicious."[51] Roman echoed similar defenses utilized by other black elites, claiming that whites were unfairly labeling the whole race based on the "lowest" examples. More than race, Roman believed class determined a person's moral and intellectual development; poor blacks were more similar in his eyes to poor whites than they were to the black elite. Class elitism was common among black Progressives, from male businessmen to black clubwomen. "Uplifting the race" was for the dual benefit of helping those less fortunate and presenting a better public image to white society.[52]

At the same time that Roman embraced class distinction between the moral and immoral, educated and ignorant, rich and poor, he called for unity of the race: "We must stand or fall together. Thank God this is true! This insures that the learned shall not despise the ignorant."[53] While Roman subscribed to a belief in the fundamental differences between middle-class and working-class blacks, he recognized that most whites did not. He then called upon whites to accept blacks into the larger community of reform, especially urging ties between black and white women involved in Progressive reform efforts.[54]

Black women's interests lay far beyond merely forging interracial ties with white women. Duty also took the form of black women's eugenic responsibility to bear and raise children, a duty that sometimes brought men and women into conflict. Black physicians stressed the important role black women played in uplifting their husbands, maintaining the health of their communities, and perpetuating the race.[55] Roman discussed the subject at length in his 1915 article, "The Negro Woman and the Health Problem." He attributed the health dangers African American communities faced to three sources, all of which he considered the responsibility of women: sexual relations, diet, and housekeeping.[56] Women's duties were to reproduce the next generation and to stand guard against sexual immorality, uncleanliness, and poor eating habits for the whole race: "woman is the determining factor in all these relations."[57] Because of women's importance in the preservation of the race, Roman addressed black women's access to sex education: "how to give woman the necessary knowledge and at the same time preserve her purity and trust, is the real woman question."[58] For Roman, purity was a higher priority than knowledge, and he adopted a decidedly anti–sex education stance. He argued, "Knowledge and goodness do not always go hand in hand. The spread of physiological knowledge without a corresponding increase in moral responsibility is of doubtful utility to mankind."[59] He further elaborated, "Our enthusiastic advocates of teaching sex-knowledge to the young, erroneously conclude that increased knowledge means increased morals, when the opposite is usually true of knowledge prematurely given."[60] Roman's reform efforts echoed the character-building white reformers. If sex education were to be provided, Roman desired that moral development should be its foremost tenet.

Dominated by Roman and other male leaders, the NMA's attitude toward women indicated a wider pattern in which the NMA, to combat pernicious sexual stereotypes and eugenic attacks, adopted a more equivocal approach to social questions.[61] For example, the birth control movement began gaining some degree of medical and social acceptance in the 1910s.[62] In contrast, the *JNMA* took a vociferous stand against the practice, citing it as dangerous not just to women's health but to the race as a whole. In one such article, NMA secretary Dr. L. L. Burwell wrote, "If we are to preserve the health of our women and check the immoral influences which arise from this practice, we must agitate against the practice." Burwell conflated contraception with abortion, calling any attempts at reproductive control "an unnatural termination." This was a common tactic for those opposing the birth control movement, forcing Margaret Sanger and other birth control advocates to spend considerable energy advocating contraception as a way to reduce women's reliance on abortion.[63] Burwell noted that contraception and abortion were harmful not just to individuals but to the race: "Woman has little knowledge of the effects on her physical being when she resorts to means of prevention. . . . There is no doubt that the frequent resorting to preventive means will destroy the health of women. . . . If the races are to be strong healthy races, we must have strong and healthy parentage."[64] Sex education would decrease interest in birth control and abortion, which would strengthen black women and the race as a whole.

Using eugenic language, the *JNMA* linked its opposition to birth control to black women's duty to bear children. Burwell cautioned blacks against using contraception, arguing that no reason could justify the dangers inherent in preventing conception for women, the race, and the nation. Black elites criticized white eugenicists for promoting genocide, while advocating positive eugenics as a way to increase black political power by expanding the educated black population. In 1913 Burwell wrote, "The fecundity, power and growth of a nation is dependent upon the fertility of woman." Implicitly tying black nationalism to the fertility of black women, Burwell tapped the well of positive eugenics.[65] Burwell warned Americans against repeating the dangerous mistakes of decadent nations like France, noting that the upper classes adopt birth control early but the lower classes slowly followed. He addressed the economic motivation some families had for limiting their offspring: "The question as to the high cost of living is an erroneous one. . . . Change of community, change of vocation and the proper exercise of thriftiness would in many cases cut down the high cost of living." His simple solution to poverty—land ownership— made his arguments more than a little specious; the path to economic security was nowhere near as simple for blacks (or whites) as Burwell suggested.[66]

The black medical establishment's stance on birth control could be read as part of the larger movement of respectability politics, challenging racist sexual stereotypes and urging blacks to control their own sexual behavior. Complicating the issue, many noted the very real problem of infant mortality among African Americans and feared that declining health exacerbated by poverty would lead to a declining population.[67] Birth control, while empowering women to make choices about their own reproductive lives, might endanger the eugenic future of the race and reinforce stereotypes of sexually promiscuous black women.

Although Burwell disapproved of contraception, he did support sex education for African American women, believing that greater knowledge would *decrease* women's interest in birth control: "medical men so often hold back reproductive facts, which would be of immense benefit to the human race in the preservation of health and the preservation of the race and nation."[68] His argument paralleled many of the white social purity advocates of the late nineteenth century, and his conclusion was the same: sex education was necessary to prepare people to make healthy and moral choices. "I think the danger that is threatening us should cause us to put aside modesty and look the facts squarely in the face and engage in our fight against it. . . . Let us do our duty."[69] Dr. Barnett M. Rhetta of Howard University Medical School wrote, "We have heard intelligent people, we have heard a few physicians say, that the problem was not how to have children, but how to keep from having them. A thing was never more wrong." Conflating contraception with abortion, he called abortionists "the greatest enemy to society, the greatest criminal[s] on earth today."[70] NMA president John A. Kenney supported sex education while rejecting birth control, stating, "All too long prudery and mock modesty have held sway at the expense of common sense while our boys and girls are drifting into bad habits, immorality, and as a consequence there is a general tendency

to racial decay. What a price to pay for silence!"[71] He hoped additional education—perhaps even in eugenics—would teach women the proper respect for
motherhood: "In biblical days sterility was a curse. Today, the tendency in some
quarters is to jeer and gibe the woman who rears a family. . . . WITH ALL THE
EMPHASIS AT MY COMMAND I SAY THAT THE WOMAN WHO IS UNABLE
OR UNWILLING TO PERFORM THE DUTIES OF WIFE AND MOTHER
SHOULD NOT MARRY."[72] Kenney's emphasis on woman's place played on
antifeminist rhetoric common among both blacks and whites. Professional
black women frequently expressed their autonomy by delaying marriage or
childrearing to pursue a career. Such choices challenged the postemancipation image of the patriarchal family that some black men desired. Some black
men defined their economic and gender privilege by their ability to keep their
wives in the home, and they resented women who refused a subordinate position in the family or refused to fulfill their reproductive duty to the race.[73]

By 1917, the language with which the NMA rejected birth control softened,
but the message was still the same. An editorial in 1917 advised, "It is well for
the public to go slow and for physicians to inform themselves fully" on the matter of birth control.[74] The *JNMA* did not include any procontraception articles
or editorials until 1918, when black Virginia physician G. Jarvis Bowens argued
that the practice might be in some cases beneficial to conserve the health of the
mother. Bowens stressed that the appropriate use of birth control varied based
on the situation, the physician's determination of the patient's worthiness, and
the eugenic results of a patient's breeding. The decision, as he saw it, rested
with the "earnest, conscientious and well meaning [*sic*] physician of today," not
the prospective mother. Several physicians quickly responded to this lukewarm
endorsement by arguing that birth control was too dangerous; one discussant
responded, "There is danger of the extinction of the human race if the essay-
ist's doctrine prevails."[75] The *JNMA* followed this debate with more anticontra-
ception pieces in the 1920s.[76] The trend of linking birth control and abortion
caused many physicians, especially those in the NMA most concerned with the
health and welfare of African American communities, to distance themselves
from contraception. Even as white physicians were beginning to embrace it,
black physicians recoiled. Duty to the race played a major role in this opinion: as violent white supremacy threatened black political power and the black
population at large, a woman's duty to maintain the race outweighed her own
personal reasons to limit her fertility. Family limitation went hand in hand with
women's autonomy and hence was threatening to some men.

Most scholars have focused on eugenics among the white population, but
the movement influenced and was influenced by nonwhites as well.[77] Some
white Progressives lauded the purported drop in black birth rates, while
blacks expressed concern. Gaining a foothold among many educated and
Progressive reformers, eugenics in both its "positive" and "negative" strains
contained significant elements of racial control. White eugenicists often

urged wealthy, native-born whites to have more children while trying to find ways to discourage or prevent racial and ethnic minorities from doing the same. The latter could be through advocating greater access to birth control devices and instruction or through more coercive methods such as forced sterilization and gender segregation for the diseased, feebleminded, or insane. Black eugenicists turned this around, arguing that middle-class and educated blacks—those most likely to have access to birth control—had a duty to the race to perpetuate or increase their numbers. On the whole, blacks recognized the dangers inherent in negative eugenics and dismissed any attempt at state control over fertility.[78] Many blacks opposed negative eugenics, fearing that whites wanted (or were already orchestrating) a decline in black birth rates in the wake of emancipation.[79]

Many middle-class African Americans advocated positive eugenics and argued that birth control was tantamount to race suicide. Rhetta's plan for a thorough sex education curriculum in high schools and colleges included teaching eugenics. Students "should be taught that the first element of attraction should be health. . . . The idea of health certificates before marriage is certainly not a bad one."[80] Rhetta argued that race suicide was the true result of the practice of contraception: "Cranks, in this country especially, have spread it that in the name of Eugenics and for the betterment of the race, the Negro in America should be silently wiped out. The consequences are that in most of the big hospitals and institutions of this country, surgical and x-ray sterilization is a common practice where the Negro is the subject." Well before the scandals of the mid-twentieth century, Rhetta addressed a practice that continued for decades: the sterilization of black women for racist purposes. He further purported that even if black women desired to be sterilized, they did not cease to be victims of the racist medical system: "too often they were willing victims." Rhetta noted the dangerous line between a woman's personal effort to control her fertility and the white medical establishment's effort to deny blacks their right to procreate.[81] Black women were caught in a matrix of power relations between white and black, male and female, and doctor and patient. Sometimes they were unknowing victims, sometimes they strategically manipulated the system for their own ends.[82] Despite the varied demands of their female patients, for the *JNMA*, building a strong race involved publicly shunning birth control thereby supporting positive eugenics.

While their debate over birth control and eugenics might have put male physicians at odds with their female patients, the *JNMA* had no such debate over the its policy on venereal disease. To fight VD and the racial stigma attached to it, black physicians first refuted white physicians' claims that venereal diseases were confined to or caused by African Americans. One contributor drew on his anecdotal experience in white hospitals, noting, "The impression has gone out that clap and gonorrhoea originated with Negroes. . . . I was connected with two hospitals this year; in one there was only one colored patient during the whole year. Fifty per cent of the people who came in gave history of having had gonorrhoea."[83] Germs, as noted by numerous physicians, did not obey the color line.[84] Contributors to the *JNMA* discussed venereal diseases as human conditions, mentioning no differences based on race. Rather, they stressed gender and morality as the determining factors in both infection and consequences.

Adding a voice from the North, black New Jersey physician Peter F. Ghee's article on chronic gonorrhea stressed the gendered aspects of the disease. Rather than emphasizing how race affected transmission or the course of the disease in black versus white bodies, Ghee compared the ways that syphilis and gonorrhea affected men and women. He mentioned infertility and impotence for men, infertility and the threat of abdominal surgeries for women. Ghee did not completely reject characterizing syphilis as a punishment, but instead of blacks being punished for their African bodies or immoral ways, he argued that men were being punished and consequently punishing their innocent wives. In Ghee's analysis, women were always the victims and men always the perpetrators. His discussants echoed Ghee's gendered analysis of VD, one emphasizing, "Innocent married women often suffer from such conditions because of the 'sins' of their husbands."[85]

It was not just women's suffering that troubled black medical professionals; both sexes suffered the ravages of venereal disease. The *JNMA* stressed prevention rather than cure, cautioning readers not to rely on treatments. Two editorials in 1911 mention the development of Salvarsan 606, an antisyphilitic drug developed two years earlier by German immunologist Paul Ehrlich.[86] Both approached the new treatment with reticence. One physician, debating the medical efficacy of the drug, cautioned, "Further observations however, have shown that its use is not unattended with dangers."[87] Another, concerned with the public's interpretation of the medication, counseled the public against quickly embracing the new drug: "The lay publications describe the new compound in such florid language that the impressionable lay mind gives credence to the idea that 606 is an infallible cure for lues [syphilis] in all of its stages. . . . In certain conditions, 606 may be positively dangerous."[88] Ghee concluded that prevention was the only effective treatment and urged, "We must advise greater chastity upon your [parents'] young men, stating the case to them plainly and frankly."[89] The emphasis on abstinence, while still providing limited information on treatment, may have allowed black physicians to emphasize respectability politics in the public sphere while still treating patients to the best of their abilities.

Providing medical and moral advice alongside other writers, black physicians played a central role in racial uplift campaigns. Physicians had their duty to impart knowledge and heal the sick just as women had their duty to bear and raise children. The information they chose to impart about sexual hygiene varied from physician to physician. Some, like Burwell and Rhetta, believed that increased knowledge would increase health without increasing contraception or sexual immorality. Others, like Roman, feared that a little knowledge would destroy innocence and encourage greater sexual curiosity. For those who agreed with Roman, the answer remained to keep children, especially girls, uninformed as long as possible.

Sexual Ignorance and Victorianism

Many middle-class blacks took as their motto the old adage that "ignorance is innocence." This may be the result of a long tradition of black women's vulnerability to sexual violence. Historian Darlene Clark Hine described black women's response to sexual oppression as dissemblance, meaning "the behavior and attitude of Black women that created the appearance of openness and disclosure but actually shielded the truth of their inner lives and selves from their oppressors." Public discussion of sexuality would not only feed white stereotypes of black women's sexuality but could potentially tear the "protective cloaks from their inner selves." Therefore, it is reasonable to suspect that many black women seeking respectability adopted greater reticence in discussing sexuality than their white counterparts.[90]

Whether through dissemblance or through Victorianism, many middle-class black women embraced a model of exaggerated purity or prudery in an effort to fend off stereotypes of black women's loose sexuality.[91] Middle-class black parents urged their daughters to present an image of extreme self-control and sexual respectability in order to combat centuries of racial prejudices.[92] Black clubwomen in the National Association of Colored Women downplayed their sexual expression.[93] In fact, they often promoted black male chivalry to protect black womanhood even though they understood the difficulty of demanding "protection" from black men, who were more likely to encounter white violence if they exercised chivalric notions of protection of home and family.[94] They hoped such middle-class sexual standards would spread to the rural and working-class population.[95] In essence, not only were the black male elites urging black women to publicly refute racist stereotypes, but they relied on women to maintain and strengthen the health and morals of the race through education, peer pressure, and sexual continence outside of marriage.[96] Aspiring black reformers recognized, however, that black women did not have to "do" anything to get labeled sexually promiscuous, and they comprehended the real dangers they faced should they fall from their very high pedestal. They had to behave as saints regardless of being labeled as sinners.

Black elites used overdrawn chivalry and sexual prudery to establish or maintain class status, what Evelyn Brooks Higginbotham termed the "politics of respectability" and what Willard Gatewood described as "the genteel performance." According to Higginbotham, black women of all classes could utilize manners, morals, and sexual purity to challenge the logic of racial subordina-tion.[97] According to Gatewood, black elites wished to present a model for emu-lation to poorer blacks, to refute racial stereotypes held by whites, and to lift up those around them as they climbed.[98] Elite men and women like John Hope and Lugenia Burns Hope conducted their public courtship (if not their pri-vate behaviors) not just in accordance with their religious and moral upbring-ing but also with an excruciating awareness that they were an example for the race, especially in matters of sexual behavior. Hope wrote to his fiancée, "I feel proud and happy and manly when I reflect that no conversation or letter, if brought to light, would cause either of us any shame. Our communication has been, with all its freedom and informality, at all times that of lady with gentle-man. We have not grown cheap."[99]

Poet Paul Laurence Dunbar and Alice Ruth Moore's courtship via corre-spondence also hinted at the demands of appearing pure. Dunbar, suffering from a heritage of abuse and a dependence on alcohol, ridiculed black women (Alice included), buying into predominant white assumptions about black women's promiscuity. Although Dunbar sexually assaulted Moore during their courtship, they still married, perhaps to maintain respectability and wash away the sin of premarital sex. He wrote his fiancée that propriety was more impor-tant than humanity.[100] Elite black men and women, like their white counter-parts, associated ladies and gentlemen with sexual continence as well as with wealth. Sexual reticence set them apart from the lower classes at the same time as they wished to uplift the masses to their higher standard. Perhaps even more than their white counterparts, elite African Americans considered the antebel-lum "cult of domesticity" gender roles a sign of refinement.[101]

Many elite black families attempted to foster sexual continence by hoping that ignorance would produce innocence. In their memoir, *Having Our Say: The Delany Sisters' First 100 Years*, Sarah and Elizabeth Delany both recalled their parents' silence about sex and reproduction. Elizabeth Delany remembered, "Our childhood years were so protected, we didn't have but the vaguest notion of what sex was. We had a neighbor who said to us once, 'You girls are so green, it's a wonder those cows don't mistake you for grass and gobble you up.'"[102] Both sisters believed this resulted from their upbringing within a prominent black family in Raleigh, North Carolina, at the turn of the twentieth century. Sarah recalled the way her father would censor Bible stories, cutting out the parts that dealt with adultery in an effort to keep his girls unaware of sex.[103] Booker T. Washington's daughter, Portia, likewise received very strict training in matters of sex and courtship. She noted both the excessive chaperonage of her youth and the internalized fear of "scandal" when, while studying in Europe, she had the opportunity to socialize with men.[104]

For African Americans, the price of sexual experimentation was not just for the individual but for the race. Historian Anastasia C. Curwood notes that courtship and marriage were both intimate relationships and representations of the race. African Americans "could not escape the effects of racial and gendered power relationships"; individual decisions could reflect upon the entire group. Sexual reticence in personal affairs and in sex education was race work as well as an individual choice. Dissemblance or silence was an understandable response to such pressures.[105]

Prescriptive literature aimed at elite young black women reflected the individual experiences of the Delany sisters and Portia Washington. One such advice manual emerged out of a series of lectures given at Tuskegee by Emma Azalia Hackley. Published in 1916, *The Colored Girl Beautiful* targeted girls in "colored boarding schools" with advice ranging from the care of hair and fingernails to the proper way to raise children. Like much of the advice literature aimed at whites, Hackley's work skated around the subject of sex education. This may be due more to her editors than to her reticence to speak frankly about the matter. Hackley wrote, "Much of the talks could not be printed because many of the questions and answers were personal," implying that the personal talks she held with girls were more forthright than a written manual could or should be.[106] This was a common theme in sex education; parents or organizations may have feared allowing forthright written material to find its way into the hands of young people, while allowing greater frankness in the talks themselves.

Hackley introduced a protofeminist brand of positive eugenics through intelligent, informed choice of marital partners when she advised black girls to "aim to marry a man mentally and physically fit to be the father of her children. An immoral, vile-tongued, untruthful or diseased father is a curse to his race. It is her duty and aim to improve racial stocks."[107] Hackley's advice did not provide much information about which diseases to avoid, but it did stress the importance of morality, truthfulness, and health to finding a prospective spouse. Hackley assumed that women must demand respectable behavior from their suitors, as men were too weak to resist a forward woman. The burden of race survival fell disproportionately on women. Black women had the duty to remain sexually pure outside of marriage, and prolific mothers once married. Hackley's advice mirrored that of physician L. L. Burwell, who agreed on the proper duties of black women, "for upon them the great responsibilities of the nation rest."[108] Embracing a public code of sexual purity, Burwell argued that women held the moral future of their people in their hands. Likewise, he implemented the language of chivalric tradition to argue for a defense of "three great principles—the purity of the maiden, the faithfulness of the wife, and the love of the mother."[109] Hackley agreed, but she presented a more autonomous image of womanhood.

Hackley's manual made obscure references to venereal disease, eugenics, prostitution, and masturbation, but repeatedly returned to the theme of propriety. Educated black girls had the duty and the honor to uplift the race through their proper behavior. She advised maintaining Gatewood's "genteel performance" even if it was all an act. She wrote, "A girl should not affect boldness. . . . One should affect modesty and purity, even if one does not feel them, that they may enhance her looks."[110] A girl did this, Hackley reminded her readers, not just for her own benefit but also to prevent men from taking liberties and to set an example to "other younger and less thoughtful girls."[111] One can see the ideas of dissemblance—a public demonstration while hiding personal feeling—in Hackley's advice.

The nearest Hackley came to addressing medical detail was in a section detailing the dangers of precocity:

> [The colored girl] should not try to be a woman too early in life, and should not marry too early. She should study her physique and her constitution. She should not permit desire and curiosity to control her good sense. Long illness, suffering, operations, and even early death may result from premature responsibility. If necessary, she should consult a physician and look the future squarely in the face.[112]

This passage hints at the dangers of early sexual experience: venereal diseases that may lead to surgery or death, and the possibility of unwanted pregnancy. It also implies that her readership seek contraception from a physician if necessary, something Hackley did not publicly endorse. Hackley's advice to affect modesty aimed at improving a woman's health, increasing her physical attractiveness, and above all fulfilling her duty to the race.[113] Hackley and other advice writers combined health, religion, and racial uplift to sell sexual restraint. Hackley's advice was not revolutionary, but her implicit feminism confronted the antifeminist leanings of many black medical professionals. Racial uplift and dissemblance did not mean female submission; Hackley subtly challenged male voices like Kenney and Roman by acknowledging the benefits of education and autonomy for black women and urging them to delay marriage and childrearing until they were ready, taking control over their own sexual destinies.[114]

Hackley's work went a step further than similar books like *On Habits and Manners*, written a generation prior for students at the Hampton Institute by teacher Mrs. M. F. Armstrong. Armstrong's work stressed purity and propriety in all social interactions and advised girls to ensure they could never fall prey to compromising situations. Armstrong, however, was a white woman, approaching the topic of etiquette for blacks from outside their community. Similarly, etiquette books like the 1891 publication, *Don't: A Book for Girls*, presented cautions for girls from a black male author.[115] Seldom could black girls find published voices from black women. The community, rather than print media, had to fill the gap.

Black Churches and Social Control

Amid demands to uplift the race, black elites often turned to religion to reduce the spread of venereal disease. Both whites and blacks made the connection between religious fervor and sexual passion. Many blacks agreed with G. Stanley Hall's analysis that adolescent passion could take the form of either sexual adventure or religious conversion, and it would be in the best interest of the community to channel people into the moral, spiritual life of Christianity. C. V. Roman wrote, "Religion itself is closely akin if not identical with [sexual] passion. Certainly, they are interchangeable." As such, they hoped that interest in religion would help to redirect sexual appetites during adolescence.

Some blacks noted the unlikelihood of assuming that religion would cure all people of all sin, observing that the same feat had not been achieved among whites. Racial stereotypes forced African Americans to play by a different, stricter set of rules when it came to sexuality. Roman acknowledged the presence of "sin" within the black community but countered, "What race is without sin? The sum proposition and prostitution and immorality are just as urgent in large cities where they are all Caucasians as in the cities where there are Negroes."[116] Joanna Moore, a white northern missionary in the rural South, also recognized the sinfulness of whites: "I have often heard it said that the colored man's religion did not keep him from lying and stealing. Does the white man's religion keep him from pride, from conformity to the world, from neglecting to send the Gospel to the heathen, and many other sins?"[117] Moore categorized certain sins as common among whites and others as common among blacks, but she recognized that religion alone did not eliminate sin. Religion and morality, while related in most people's minds, were not synonymous. Early twentieth-century African American historian Carter G. Woodson wrote, "It has been said that the Negroes do not connect morals with religion. The historian would like to know what race or nation does such a thing. Certainly the whites with whom the Negroes have come into contact have not done so." Woodson argued that since whites held a near monopoly over "expertise," they were able to teach both whites and blacks about the Negro's ostensibly inferior position, therefore rationalizing the use of discrimination, neglect, and violence to maintain white supremacy.[118]

The "white monopoly" first lost its hold in the realm of religion. Black churches developed strong and independent institutional power by the early twentieth century and provided infrastructural support to improve both health and morality among their members and the surrounding community. Ministers and women's organizations within various denominations employed creative strategies to counter white stereotypes and to discourage what they considered immoral behavior among the "unsaved." Churches provided alternatives to the red light district and the saloon, including recreational facilities, classes, reading rooms, and clubs. Some took more confrontational methods, such as holding open-air worship services in the middle of red light districts.[119] Both health and social advice literature, written by and for African Americans, usually stressed the religious imperative to remain sexually pure and to keep sex a sacred marital act.[120]

Despite black organization and activity to promote these ends, many whites dismissed the idea that religious moral education could work for blacks. They argued that character building, the cornerstone of the white sex education movement, did not apply to blacks, who lacked the basic religious, cultural, and even physical elements of character. According to white physician William Lee Howard, "The Caucasian as a race is moral; the African as a distinct race is not immoral, he is unmoral, and no amount of education or training is going to change a non-existent element." He equated black religion with "voodoo worship," camp meetings, extreme emotionalism, and superstition, arguing that black churches, despite their claims to Christianity, were really just rituals of savagery.[121] James Bardin concurred, writing, "It is . . . very hard to induce [the Negro] to sacrifice his own interests for the benefit of others. And he has seldom shown evidence of any feeling of responsibility toward the community in which he lives."[122] Since racist whites believed blacks lacked the capacity for moral development, they dismissed the black church as useless.

White sociologists doubted the claims made by black middle-class reformers. Howard Odum refuted any claim to moral superiority by black ministers, women's clubs, or schools, arguing that black women were immoral and that even male preachers could not be expected to uphold morality for themselves or for their communities. Indeed, Odum doubted that the black church served any socially useful purpose: "The function of the Negro Church is rather to give expression and satisfaction to social and religious emotions than to direct moral conduct."[123] Odum and Howard used similar phrases, describing blacks as "unmoral" rather than "immoral"—lacking entirely the capacity for moral development and therefore beyond the reach of education, reform, or uplift.

Anthropologists and psychologists in the Progressive Era saw race as a "seamless mix of biology and culture," so that both physical and cultural attributes were labeled race related. Black religious belief, in whites' view, had as much to do with black bodies as it did with black minds or souls.[124] Even when white critics seemed willing to assume that blacks were sincere in their religious expression, they doubted the very morality of that religion. William H. Holloway, an educator in Alabama, argued that "more than any other people, perhaps, [the Negro] takes his religion seriously." He elaborated that rather than helping blacks resist sexual urges and stay healthy, black religion actually encouraged them to indulge. "The church, which was and still is the center and controlling influence of all his activities . . . has no doubt helped to intensify the immoral, which its purpose is to rectify and cure." Blacks sinned, he argued, because their religion encouraged it.[125]

"Expert" voices continued to denigrate the black church as merely a source of amusement or excitement well into the twentieth century.[126] Even writers sympathetic to the cause of racial equality distanced themselves from what they saw as the moral handicap left over from slavery. White Baptist missionary Joanna Moore declared that black religious institutions failed to make a change in their flock's behavior. She blamed this largely on the legacy of slavery, which she believed destroyed black men's adherence to monogamy and willingness to protect black women's honor. She also blamed black ministers, who she argued were ignorant of or misinterpreted the Bible. Moore's disappointment was tempered by her optimism for the future, believing that every year away from slavery would bring blacks closer to the proper Christian standards.[127] E. Franklin Frazier, a black sociologist in the mid-twentieth century, accepted some of the ideas put forth by white missionaries like Moore: "The churches undertook as organizations to censure unconventional and immoral sex behaviour and to punish by expulsion sex offenders and those who violated the monogamous *mores*. But it was impossible to immediately change the loose and unregulated sex and family behavior among a people lacking the institutional basis of European sexual *mores*. Very often the church had to tolerate or accommodate themselves to sexual irregularities."[128] Criticism from generally sympathetic voices such as Moore's, as well as the blatant racism of critics such as Odum and Howard, eroded the vision of the black church as a useful tool in character building. Coping with denigration by whites and even by some black social scientists, African American churches hesitated to provide any sex education beyond the doctrine of purity.

The effort to stop the spread of venereal disease in the Progressive Era highlighted tangled relationships among race, class, and gender. Southern white physicians attempted to create a discourse of disease that focused on the anatomical failings of African Americans, stressing the futility of either education or treatment to save the diseased race. By stressing biological differences between the races, whites lumped all blacks into a common category. Black physicians and other professionals, battling for respect and recognition both within their communities and from whites, attempted to refashion deviant sexuality as a class problem rather than a race problem. Wary of the negative eugenic thread prominent in contemporary medical literature, black elites promoted positive eugenics and urged their audiences, especially black women, to advance their moral and educational opportunities, avoid venereal disease, and improve the race. Black male medical professionals were publicly reticent about sex education and tended to reject birth control entirely, in order to countermand destructive sexual stereotypes and the threat of race suicide. Women authors often employed a more evasive approach, practicing dissemblance while possibly opening the door for greater female sexual autonomy. Efforts at quarantine and avoidance helped solidify segregation in the South, as white medical experts portrayed blacks as morally depraved and physically diseased. African American men and women challenged the so-called expertise of white physicians, creating their own curriculum in the constrained space of racial segregation. However, segregation did not prevent the spread of venereal disease on either side of the color line nor the transmission of germs across the color line. With the advent of World War I, the nation would begin to recognize the VD problem not solely as a racial problem but as a national threat.

Chapter Five

Sex Education in the American Expeditionary Force

Dr. George Walker, a colonel in the Army Medical Corps, published a report in 1922 about venereal disease and sexuality during World War I. In it, Walker raised the specter of dangerous "French" influences on the more than four million men who had served their country during the war.[1] Among these was the spread of what he called "sex abnormalities," what we today would call oral sex. Walker feared that these new sexual activities gained popularity among the less-experienced or less-adventurous American doughboys, causing "a subtle state of demoralization that is far more dangerous to society as it is at present constructed . . . than mere immorality could ever be."[2] It seemed many American soldiers during World War I received plenty of sex education. But what were they learning and from whom? World War I marked a high point in the history of sex education, as the military took an active role in teaching it for the increased health, efficiency, and morality of its soldiers.

At the turn of the twentieth century, Americans were feeling the concomitant pressures of two major social and ideological impulses: imperialism abroad and Progressivism at home. The two often contradicted one another in their beliefs and realities. Many Progressives feared that a large American empire might distract policy makers from problems at home or add new problems to an already overtaxed society.[3] In 1900, after defeating the Spanish in Cuba and the Philippines during the Spanish-American War, the United States entered into a long occupation of the Philippine Islands, a new American protectorate. The imperialistic militarism exhibited by such actions aroused the anger of anti-imperialists at home. Muckraking exposés highlighted the contradictions inherent in American imperialism. Some factions of Progressives and anti-imperialists alike considered the Philippine incursion a violation of American ideals. They complained that American "civilization," through the influence of the American military presence, degraded rather than uplifted the native population.

The reaction stateside to action abroad signaled a substantial change in American attitudes toward military life, prostitution, and the role of the government in moral protection. The Chicago *New Voice*, a leading prohibitionist newspaper, sent a journalist to report on conditions in Manila in 1900. The Chicago reporter, William B. Johnson, wrote, "Far more of our boys who are lying there met their death through bad women and drink than through the bullets of the Filipinos. Five hundred American soldiers were recently exhumed from this field and sent to the States, mostly victims of drink and lust."[4] Follow-up articles chided the US military for instituting regulated prostitution abroad, a policy that already had failed at home.[5] Henry B. Blackwell, coeditor of the *Woman's Journal*, commented that Johnson's report "discloses the shameful fact that the State Regulation of Vice, which exists nowhere in this country, having been abolished years ago in St. Louis by an uprising of the good women and men of that city, has been introduced, and is being openly enforced by the army authorities in Manila."[6] To Blackwell and others, this report confirmed the immorality of imperialism, the dangers of a militaristic state, and the subsequent need for woman suffrage to bring a moral compass to national politics.

The outrage Progressives and anti-imperialists expressed over regulated prostitution surprised some military leaders. Prostitution near military bases was not universally accepted, but much of the military either approved of or ignored it. Prostitutes and camp followers had accompanied the US Army on numerous campaigns and became an accepted part of military life.[7] Yet between 1900 and 1917, when the United States entered World War I, the government restyled its policies and assumptions regarding prostitution and sexual necessity. In the throes of Progressive reform, the American public had begun refuting the idea that men required sexual activity to stay healthy. Reformers moved toward a single standard of sexual morality and an awareness of the dangers of venereal diseases not just to individuals but to the nation as a whole. Sexual education was central to the goals of Progressive reformers, and the military provided a venue to accomplish their mission.

This chapter argues that World War I provided a catalyst, opportunity, and turning point for the American sex education movement. Progressive efforts at establishing broad-based sex education for young Americans, which met considerable resistance everywhere it had been introduced, took center stage as the United States became embroiled in a world war. Sex education, especially when targeted at soldiers, went from being of questionable benefit to being a matter of national security. As a result, in 1917 and 1918 the military and government increased their role in guiding the morality of soldiers and civilians. The federal government formed an infrastructure, in cooperation with the American Social Hygiene Association and other social hygiene reformers, enforced the policing of sexual behavior in the military and demanded medical treatment for those who exposed themselves to venereal infection. They eventually developed the "American Plan," which included wholesome recreation, sex education information for soldiers, and medical treatment for those infected. The American Plan received credit for reducing VD rates among American soldiers and for changing public opinion about sex education.

Encountering the Enemy, Intimately

The concern over military cleanliness can be traced from the Philippine occupation to the Punitive Expedition into Mexico in 1916, and eventually to France in World War I. Military officials expressed deep concern over the apparent "uncleanliness" of soldiers in the Philippines, which scholar Aaron Belkin notes marks the beginning of a transition from a nineteenth-century military ideal of rough and rugged masculinity to a masculinity marked by self-control and discipline. Military leaders continuously complained that their men were mired in "filth" in the Philippines, which served to explain the high rates of venereal disease. However, the federal government did not yet take seriously that the disease vector did not flow only from the Filipinos to the Americans but rather in both directions.[8] Rather, tropical climates and nonwhite women seemed to be to blame, in keeping with white medical assumptions.

While still in the Philippines, the American military began taking tentative steps toward coping with venereal disease. Ironically, it was not through Progressive antiprostitution efforts that studies of the problem first emerged but rather through the temperance movement. In 1901, the Army outlawed the sale of beer and light wines at army canteens, to the applause of prohibitionists. Military motives did not end with curbing drink. Officials connected the abolition of the canteen to controlling spread of venereal disease, proclaiming a link between alcohol and sexual transgression. Other military officials challenged this view. In a medical corps report, published in June 1917, retired medical officer Colonel Louis M. Maus wrote:

> Following the abolishment of the army beer canteen [in 1901], a large number of prominent people in civil life, including many physicians, members of altruistic societies, newspaper men, and even members of the clergy, endeavored to prove that the abrogation of the beer feature of the canteen was largely responsible for the increase of the venereal incidence in the Army, and for years industriously endeavored to secure a repeal of the law.[9]

Maus argued that the Canteen Act actually increased soldiers' visits to houses of prostitution, since it drove them off base to find alcohol, often to saloons in red light districts.[10] Maus pointed out that the VD rate was high throughout the early years of the twentieth century, peaking in 1911 at just over 185 per 1,000. He blamed this increase on the lack of a coherent military policy: "Although medical inspections and venereal prophylaxes had occupied the attention of medical officers since the Spanish War [of 1898], these important sanitary measures never received official recognition from the War Department until . . . 1912" when biweekly venereal inspections were authorized.[11] Many commanders had experimented with regulated prostitution and venereal prophylaxis since the turn of the century. All their measures fell short because the military failed to take a firm, uniform policy and enforce it across the entire service or to consider the multiple factors causing women to turn to prostitution.

Arguing that no single solution could eliminate the problem, Maus praised the "liberal and progressive" multifaceted suggestions for new military policy advocated by Surgeon General George Henry Torney.[12] In 1909, Torney issued an office circular recommending a four-point plan for reducing the high rates of venereal disease in the Army. First, he encouraged "wholesome recreation" at military posts to decrease the draw of red light districts. Second, he recommended sex education be provided to soldiers through lectures and personal advice that discussed prostitution, VD, and the dangers of contagion to not only the self but to innocent wives and children at home. Third, he declared the importance of regular physical examinations to detect VD early in its course. Fourth, he advocated preventive medical treatment for those who still visited prostitutes.[13]

In the years immediately following 1909, the government remained hesitant to implement any of these measures. Noting fear of public opinion, Maus wearily concluded, "I will state here, that the War Department felt it necessary to guard the Government from the criticism of the moral societies and press of the country, which were liable to have been aroused at that time."[14] Public opinion evidently played a major role in military policy. Maus concluded, "Each year brings us nearer the goal of public and frank discussion of these great problems, which are responsible for three-fourths of human degeneracy and wretchedness."[15] Despite the continued concern expressed by medical officers like Maus and Torney, real change did not occur until concerns about military efficiency brought the subject to light in 1916.

The Punitive Expedition into Mexico, 1916

A year before the United States entered World War I, the army experienced a test of its soldiers' fortitude: warfare with Mexico. In March 1916, Francisco "Pancho" Villa led an attack across the border into New Mexico, prompting Woodrow Wilson to send troops to the region. The pursuit of Villa, led by General John J. Pershing, commenced in fits and starts along the borderlands and into the Mexican interior. After the expedition set up its base camp in Mexico, the troops settled in for a long wait, trying to determine which action to take while the Army considered its options. Looming war in Europe reduced the priority placed on the Mexican Punitive Expedition. Along with uncertainty came idle time, creating a problem for Pershing and his staff. Idle time invited lapses in discipline and training.

The American troops found easy access to prostitutes while stationed in northern Mexico. Pershing and his staff, concerned about morality and military efficiency, debated how to handle the influx of prostitutes to their base camp and the subsequent increase in VD-related sick time. Pershing decided to take the suggestion of his advisors and continue the unofficial army policy of regulation. The general assigned one of his medical officers to be health inspector, set up a restricted red light district, and set the standard fee at two dollars. VD rates declined almost immediately, and the general wrote to a colleague, "The establishment was necessary and has proved the best way to handle a difficult problem." Pershing also noted that there seemed to be little concern from the United States about his move, which was in keeping with previous military policy.[16]

Pershing underestimated the response of the American public. Since reports of immorality from the Spanish-American War fifteen years before, Progressive reformers routinely investigated any unseemly policies that might influence soldiers' morality, refusing to leave it all in the hands of the military chain of command. During the Punitive Expedition, both the federal government and independent organizations sent representatives to the Mexican border to observe soldiers' conditions. What they found did not reassure the Wilson administration and the reform-minded public.[17]

Raymond B. Fosdick, a Progressive activist who had studied the white slave traffic in New York City under the auspices of the Rockefeller Foundation, was asked by the War Department to visit the border camps and provide an eye-witness, expert account of conditions. He reported to Secretary of War Newton Baker that prostitution was on the rise, with each town enlarging its red light districts and women from both sides of the border flocking to camps. According to Baker, "Meanwhile, the venereal disease rates were soaring. The difficulty of the situation, as I told the Secretary of War, was that no uniform policy in relation to this situation had been developed by the army, and the ideas and attitudes of the divisional and camp commanders showed the widest variation. Most of the regular army officers . . . shrugged it off as a hopeless problem."[18] In other words, without a clear stance by the military itself, commanders merely implemented the method they found best to cope with the situation. This meant regulation of a red light district in some areas, restriction in others. For many, it meant ignoring the problem altogether.

Fosdick's report recommended that the War Department produce a definite policy and require troop commanders to comply with restriction "in the interest of the efficiency of its troops against the unrestrained excesses of prostitution and the saloon." He proposed a two-pronged plan: first, military and civilian officials must work together to close down the brothels and deny access to prostitutes. If a town failed to cooperate, the government should remove the troops. Second, according to Fosdick, the government had a responsibility to provide alternative entertainment and recreation to the soldiers. He observed:

> I remembered the five thousand troops encamped just across the railroad tracks from Columbus, New Mexico, and the way they used to come to town

every evening—almost in a body—to escape the monotony of camp life. And what did they find when they came to town? There were no moving picture shows and no pool tables; there was no place where they could read or write letters; there were no homes to which they could go. . . . The only attraction in town was a few disreputable saloons and a red light district. These institutions had the field to themselves; there was nothing to compete with them.[19]

Fosdick recommended policies that would both discourage immoral behavior and provide alternatives for the soldiers. To do this, the federal government would take a far more active role in morally policing their soldiers than ever before.

The YMCA, just beginning to invest time and energy into social work among the soldiers on the border, immediately assisted with Fosdick's plan. In June 1916, George A. Reeder of the YMCA completed a report of conditions along the border, stating that the "moral risks of the troops are greater than the Association has ever faced before. Under the monotony of military camp life, in a most trying climate, the temptations to which thousands of young men away from home will be subjected are very great."[20] The YMCA echoed the concerns of the military that soldiers lacked alternative recreation to keep them from brothels. Reflecting medical men's association of hot climates with uncontrolled sexuality, reformers feared that the inhospitable climate and the menacing presence of "tens of thousands of Mexican women" would prove disastrous for the men.[21] Reformers thus categorized the enemy by race as well as by gender.

During the late nineteenth and early twentieth centuries, race- and class-based stereotypes damaged relations between the United States and Mexico. White Americans held on to historical ideas of superiority while experiencing a newer, perhaps more virulent, feeling of hygienic contamination from Mexicans in the borderlands. Many white Anglos saw Mexicans as dirty and diseased and a medical and social threat to nearby whites. The risk of contamination helped justify segregation, antimiscegenation, or even "quarantine" between white Anglos and Mexicans or Mexican Americans.[22] Whites assigned moral values to nonwhites, differentiating them from whites. Whites often believed that Mexicans, like other nonwhite peoples, were morally corrupt and lacked the sense of propriety that whites had.[23] These attitudes did not always discourage interaction between the races. White moral rhetoric helped created a fantasy of Mexican women as erotic, sensuous, and voluptuous.[24] Racial stereotypes of Mexican women's sexuality harked back to the same theories many whites held about black women, which served to justify white dalliance with black prostitutes and mistresses, or even sexual violence against nonwhite women. Likewise, whites occasionally identified Mexican blood with promiscuity and criminality and linked Mexicans with "savages" and Native Americans.[25] Stereotypes paradoxically both discouraged and justified interracial sex. Women of color were thought, by the "tropical" nature of their race as well as by the moral laxity of their culture, to invite or instigate sexual relations with white men. The soldiers along the border could look down on these women as inferior beings but still be forgiven for purchasing sex from them.[26]

White Anglos held similar stereotypes concerning the prevalence of venereal disease among Mexicans and African Americans. Dr. W. H. Blodgett of Mercedes, Texas, echoed many white southern doctors' assumptions about race determining disease: "The thing most dreaded by the army commanders and the army doctors outside the bullets of the enemy is venereal diseases. And this is especially true on the border where the lower class of Mexicans who form a large per cent of the population are infected with venereal disorders."[27] Blodgett assumed an almost universal contamination of the poorer Mexican population.[28]

YMCA agent and medical doctor Max Exner spent seven weeks in 1917 among the troops along the border and in Mexico, visiting several camps and reporting not just on VD rates but also on the general state of recreation, law enforcement, and the red light districts. Exner, a respected figure in ASHA and the sex education movement, questioned the inevitability of prostitution, the very assumption upon which the military policy of regulated prostitution rested. He stated, "I rarely met an officer who did not take for granted that prostitution could not or should not be abolished. They assumed that it is necessary for the contentment and well-being of the men, or, at least, that it is inevitable."[29] One high-ranking cavalry officer with whom he spoke argued, "You must remember that we have among the troops men of a very low order— men with little brains and powerful passions. If prostitution were not provided, these men would disobey orders, go to Mexican villages and get mixed up with the women and thereby possibly bring on war."[30] The cavalry officer implied that class played a role in whether a man could control his sexual instincts; the men of a "very low order," while necessary to fill out military recruitment, raised problems of discipline and control.

Exner noted the long tradition of assuming that sexual indulgence was both medically necessary for men's health and socially necessary to maintain military discipline. He then structured his entire report to contradict these assumptions, noting the drawbacks to prostitution from medical, moral, and disciplinary perspectives: "It is a matter of history that prostitution follows the army. In all the European armies at the present time vice and its consequences constitute one of the most serious, if not the most serious, of army problems."[31] He argued that the experience along the Mexican border proved that prostitution was neither desirable nor inevitable. This odd assumption was especially worrying because it affected the character development of soldiers "in their adolescent years." Exner built upon theories of adolescent development and the need to educate, with a strong dose of morality, those suffering from the throes of the turbulent sex instinct: "If there is ever a time when the man needs every possible moral support and influence to steady him and keep him true to his best self, this is the time."[32] The soldiers on the border, lacking a proper education in sexual matters and suffering in a harsh and lonely climate, needed help to refuse the evil influences about them.

Race played a significant role in the way the military addressed prostitution along the Mexican border. Exner's report assigned letters to specific camps to disguise their location. For each, he noted the presence of vice districts, often identifying them by the race of prostitutes available. One camp actually went so far as to close down the Mexican houses of prostitution in an effort to slow the spread of VD, while allowing the whites and blacks to continue business.[33]

Exner's report urged the medical community to "refute the contention of so large a proportion of army officers that sexual indulgence is necessary for the contentment of the men." Camp H demonstrated that military efficiency could exist apart from easily accessible prostitution; that camp benefited not from repressive measures but from its geographic isolation and lack of transportation infrastructure—the men could not physically get to the prostitutes. Camp I was a large camp, situated near existing saloons and red light districts. Exner praised how Camp I's commander "suppressed both absolutely with an iron hand and never relaxed his vigilance."[34] Despite the harsh crackdown, the soldiers of Camp I remained orderly, disciplined, and efficient while stationed there. Exner noted how the men stationed there developed a pride in their moral reputation: "Many of the men said to me, 'Oh, we have a clean bunch here.'"[35]

Exner also reported that many of the soldiers were infected with venereal diseases *before* their arrival in Mexico, and thus they posed as much, if not more, of a threat to the local prostitutes than vice versa. This conclusion would later be confirmed when draftees in World War I took their medical exams. Whether the disease traveled from soldier to civilian or vice versa, the conditions contributed to a high rate of disease in both groups.[36] Exner's answer: the military must support a policy of repression rather than regulation, and the municipal and military authorities must work together to provide a "reasonably wholesome environment" for the soldiers. It was the national duty to value good health and clean living as well as efficiency, through restrictive measures, sex education, and (if all else failed) medical prophylaxis.

Exner concluded that the examples of Camp I's repression and Camp H's lack of access demonstrated the benefits of a prostitution-free environment. It was not only possible but also necessary and desirable. "Whenever I suggested the possibility of attacking not only the results of prostitution, but prostitution itself, I was looked upon as 'too idealistic,' or as a dreaming, unpractical reformer."[37] He wished to demonstrate the connections between moral ideals and military efficiency. In this way, Exner stood against the practical compromise that military leaders like Pershing, however reluctantly, espoused. Exner agreed with Fosdick, arguing that an idealistic policy could be feasible if given the right support and resources. This was what he wished to see writ large in America's future military actions.[38]

Widespread press coverage by nationally known figures like Exner and Fosdick influenced the policy adopted during the Punitive Expedition. By the time real progress had been made regarding prostitution and venereal disease along the Mexican border, however, it became apparent that the problem of keeping the army "fit to fight" was larger than a border skirmish. US involvement in the European war seemed imminent by January 1917, influencing a decision to evacuate American troops from Mexico by spring. Exner and Fosdick would take their findings from Mexico and apply them on a grand scale as the nation mobilized for war. Fosdick wrote to Secretary Baker, "The situation had improved on the Mexican border. . . . The cribs are closed, at least for the moment, and so are most of the fly-by-night saloons on the roads to the camps. But you and I have had enough experience in city government to know that this *verboten* approach isn't going to accomplish a great deal. It's *part* of the answer, but not the whole answer."[39] Fosdick returned to Washington to discuss the lessons of the Punitive Expedition and how they might use those lessons productively in America's next big challenge: global war.

World War I and the American Plan

On April 6, 1917, President Woodrow Wilson asked Congress for a declaration of war. After a long period of deteriorating neutrality, this hardly came as a surprise. What was surprising was the way in which the US government would radically alter its policy toward prostitution, sex education, and venereal disease. Secretary Baker and President Wilson remained staunch in their refusal to yield to the "French" plan (or Pershing's practice) of regulated prostitution. In fact, in one of the more telling exchanges of cultural differences among the Allies, French premier Georges Clemenceau criticized the American policy of repression and suggested that he could help establish clean brothels for the doughboys. Upon receiving this response, Fosdick told Baker, "For God's sake, Raymond, don't show this to the President or he'll stop the war."[40] A war to end all wars, or a war to preserve democracy, was a battle worth fighting, but not if it jeopardized the morality of the soldiers asked to fight.

Baker and Fosdick had already begun translating the lessons of the Mexican border campaign into the Army's network of training camps. Woodrow Wilson endorsed their efforts: "the Federal Government has pledged its word that as far as care and vigilance can accomplish the result, the men committed to its charge will be returned to their homes and communities which so generously gave them with no scars except those won in honorable warfare."[41] Wilson thus promised his support to the creation of a military that would protect its soldiers' souls as well as their bodies.[42] Secretary of War Newton Baker echoed those words, stating, "I want them to have an armor made up of a set of social habits replacing those of their homes and communities . . . a moral and intellectual armor for their protection overseas."[43] Baker wanted not just to preserve the morals of the American home but to improve upon them.[44] Reformers envisioned the World War I training camps as an ideal Progressive laboratory for training the troops in military efficiency, patriotism, Americanism, and middle-class morality.[45] Central to this goal was an all-encompassing program for VD eradication and sex education. In contrast to the French and former US strategy of regulated prostitution, Fosdick, Baker, and other influential figures developed the American Plan, aimed at making the American Expeditionary Force (AEF) the cleanest, fittest, and most moral army in the world.

It took less than two weeks for the War Department to establish the Commission on Training Camp Activities (CTCA), headed by Raymond Fosdick, in an effort to change the moral and physical health of the American Expeditionary Force.[46] The CTCA, in conjunction with the Interdepartmental Social Hygiene Board, the US Public Health Service, and ASHA, instituted the so-called American Plan to combat venereal disease in the Army and Navy. Rejecting regulated prostitution, Fosdick wished to combine medical treatment, education, wholesome recreation, and law enforcement to improve the health and morality of the AEF. This four-point plan was reminiscent of Surgeon General Torney's 1909 plan, except this time it had backing. The plan's four divisions would each contribute to the development of a well-informed, patriotic soldier who would embrace sexual abstinence out of knowledge of its consequences for his body, his soul, and his country.[47]

The American Plan, in name and in purpose, indicated how the US government saw its work as a break from the pragmatic attitude of the French and other European powers and America's own military history. The literature it produced reflected a belief in American exceptionalism. Educational materials aimed at soldiers repeated statistics on various European armies' troubles with venereal diseases, one admonishing Americans to "see that the sad experience of European nations would not be repeated in our country."[48] By differentiating moral America from decadent Europe, the military reinforced the concept of chastity as a patriotic duty. A news bulletin from the YMCA National War Work Council applauded the military's efforts to both lecture to soldiers and provide useful pamphlets on sex education. The YMCA urged these efforts, stating, "Such work as this is indispensable if the American army is to escape the pit into which so many of the troops of other nations have fallen in this war."[49] Pride in self and country united, as soldiers were urged to demonstrate their patriotism: Charles Larned Robinson of the YMCA told the soldiers, "You Americans are going to show the world how a soldier should fight, and if necessary how he should die. Show the world how a soldier should live."[50]

The nation needed sex education more than ever, and public opinion had turned a corner under the stress of military necessity. Dr. R. Hooker of ASHA noted that US entry into World War I resulted in both the VD "problem made acute" and a "growing responsiveness of public opinion to progressive legislation and administration."[51] Fosdick wrote later that his work on the Mexican border with Newton Baker greatly influenced his work with the CTCA. Baker told him, "We cannot afford to draft them into a demoralizing environment. It will be your job to see that their surroundings in the camps are not allowed to be less stimulating and worthy than the environment in their home communities."[52] To ensure the sanctity of training camps, the federal government created "white zones," areas in which no alcohol or prostitution was permitted, surrounding military installations. There may have been racial overtones to the term, since often the establishment of a "white zone" practically meant the eviction of African American and Mexican American women who were assumed to be prostitutes, as well as pushing actual prostitutes into adjacent nonwhite neighborhoods.[53] The selective draft law of April 28, 1917, gave Wilson and Baker the power to regulate and prohibit saloons and houses of ill fame. Baker justified this intrusion into civilian life as part of the war effort and thus an emergency measure: "we cannot allow these young men, most of whom will have been drafted to service, to be surrounded by a vicious and demoralizing environment, nor can we leave anything undone which will protect them from unhealthy influence, and crude forms of temptation."[54]

Progressive reformers who had the ear of the president considered regulated houses of prostitution to be passé. They publicized their viewpoints, backed with sociological evidence from the Mexican expedition, and convinced even the military hierarchy. Dr. George Walker, a colonel in the Army Medical Corps, praised General Pershing's change of heart from regulation to prevention, writing that both the European experience and the experience of soldiers in training camps within the United States would demonstrate a "continuation of the work he had done in the same direction among the men of his army in Mexico." By July 1918, "the Commander-in-Chief had completely changed his opinion and was firmly convinced that houses of prostitution should not be tolerated."[55] The federal government was now ready to take action both to provide sex education to its soldiers and to treat or punish those who put themselves at risk for sexually transmitted diseases.

Medical Treatment

One of the most controversial aspects of the American Plan was the establishment of a standard of medical treatment for soldiers who were exposed to or infected with venereal diseases. The controversy split the tenuous alliance between purity advocates and medical hygiene reformers.[56] The military, the medical establishment, and the general public debated whether the promise of treatment would grant soldiers a license to be immoral. The Navy had introduced chemical prophylaxis in 1908, but few of the units made it compulsory.

At a chemical prophylactic station, a medical attendant would instruct a soldier to clean his genitals with soap and water, followed by a bichloride solution. The attendant would then treat the urethra and advise the soldier to avoid urination or genital contact for several hours. Medical personnel recommended performing the treatment within three hours of exposure to infection to increase the chance of success.[57] Use varied, depending on the attitude of the commanding and medical officers in each unit and the availability of stations and supplies. Pocket-sized "K-Packets," which contained a chemical solution that men could inject themselves with after intercourse, also served to decrease the incidence of infection. In his study of venereal disease in the US military, Walker reported that by 1909 the VD rates were falling in the Navy from 156 per 1,000 to 76 per 1,000, a change he attributed to the introduction of chemical prophylaxis.[58]

The Navy's experimentation with prophylaxis halted when President Wilson appointed Josephus Daniels secretary of the Navy in March of 1913. Daniels saw chemical prophylaxis as "an invitation to sin," and he refused to sanction any plan for prophylaxis. He also prohibited K-packets on Navy ships. Daniels demonstrated his attitude in his 1915 letter to commanding officers:

> The spectacle of an officer or hospital steward calling up boys in their teens as they are going on leave and handing over these "preventative packets" is abhorrent to me. It is equivalent to the government advising these boys that it is right and proper for them to indulge in an evil which perverts their morals. I would not permit a youth in whom I was interested to enlist in a service that would thus give virtual approval to disobeying the teachings of his parents and the dictates of the highest moral code. You may say that the ideal raised is too high and we need not expect young men to live up to the ideal of continence. If so, I cannot agree. It is a duty we cannot shirk to point to the true ideal, to chastity, to a single standard of morals for men and women.[59]

He rejected both preexposure protection and postexposure prophylaxis in the Navy. He described condoms as "propaganda which tends to condone the sin of illicit sexual intercourse and engender in the young men of the Navy the belief that they have been provided with a method or means which will diminish the danger of unlawful or sinful misconduct."[60] For him, his duty as secretary of the Navy was to protect not just sailors' lives but also their souls. Daniels wanted the military to be a training ground for moral manhood, functioning in loco parentis for young recruits, and he, the father figure, took the lead as moral arbiter. His quest for a predictable social hierarchy fit well into the modern, Progressive notion of an orderly military life, even as he retained Victorian purity attitudes.[61]

Personally, Daniels espoused the social purity movement that had dominated sex education for a generation before the war, particularly its call for a single standard of morality.[62] Like his friend and fellow Wilson appointee,

Williams Jennings Bryan, Daniels had taught Sunday school, favored prohibition, and embraced evangelical Christianity.[63] He believed that the single standard should be attained by raising men to the level of chastity society expected of women. This idea meshed with the changing opinions of medical experts, who recently had contradicted the popular idea that sexual indulgence was necessary to preserve male health. Daniels' views did not mesh well with the military's traditional laissez-faire attitude toward sexual morality, however, or with many soldiers' personal experiences. As demonstrated by the Philippine and Mexican experience, Army officers usually looked the other way when it came to soldiers' involvement with prostitution and sexual dalliance.

Naval officers may have disagreed with Daniels, but few risked defying him. A resolute advocate of chemical prophylaxis, Colonel Walker of the Medical Corps wrote disapprovingly, "His inflexible, prejudicial attitude discouraged most of the medical officers from taking any interest whatsoever in prophylactic stations on ships." Walker reported that the secretary's attitude trickled down to those under his command, who feared "getting into trouble if they said much about this treatment."[64]

Daniels' stance against prophylaxis dismayed Fosdick and Baker as well. Fosdick remarked at the beginning of the war that the Navy had higher rates of disease than the Army, and he blamed this on Daniels: "I was confident that the discrepancy was due to the Navy's failure to install the system of medical prophylaxis after exposure—a system which had been enforced in the Army for several years. My presentation of the case to Daniels, however, got me nowhere."[65] Fosdick had to come up with a way around the secretary of the Navy if he wished to fully implement the American Plan:

> One day Daniels said to me, as if in despair, for I was pressing him hard, and so were the Navy doctors: "I wish I didn't have to make the decision." A few days later he left on an inspection trip, and [Franklin Delano] Roosevelt was Acting Secretary of the Navy. I immediately took the situation up with him and told him of Daniel's remark. "In that case," he said, "I'll make the decision myself," and he signed the order [to provide prophylaxis]. Its effect on the venereal disease rate was soon apparent.[66]

The VD rates decreased quickly. Fosdick later speculated that Daniels felt relieved to have the decision taken out of his hands. His moral ideology had boxed him into a corner as he encountered pressure from the War Department and from within the Navy Department. Fosdick and Roosevelt solved the dilemma without forcing Daniels to step back from his beliefs.

With the Navy joining ranks, the military set forth a plan for bimonthly health inspections and the establishment of chemical prophylactic stations. On July 3, 1917, Pershing passed General Order #6, providing for Army prophylactic stations "at convenient places to be determined by the commanding officer and the surgeon" and bimonthly venereal inspections for soldiers by a medical officer.[67] Article 2955 of the Navy Regulations stated, "All men upon return-ing to their ships or station shall be given opportunity to admit exposure to infection with venereal disease if such exposure shall have occurred, and all such men shall receive early medical prophylactic treatment and continued treatment until cured if prophylaxis fails." It further stipulated that men who refused to seek treatment and acquired a venereal infection would be subject to court-martial and segregation from their unit at home and abroad.[68]

The medical branch of the War Department declared the chemical prophy-laxis, if properly administered within the allotted time frame of three hours, was 99.6 percent effective in preventing venereal infection.[69] The propaganda provided to soldiers told a different story, one more grounded in the moral ambivalence surrounding chemical prophylaxis than in hard science. Pam-phlets first and foremost stressed abstinence, but they recognized that it would not deter all sexual indulgence. One notice to soldiers warned, "If, in spite of this warning, you do have illicit sexual intercourse, go at once to the regi-mental infirmary for early treatment, and the men there will do their best to prevent you from becoming infected. The best that can be done to prevent infection still leaves risk enough and you cannot rely upon this treatment to make it safe for you to stay with women." The pamphlet then reported that reg-ulations required a soldier to report within eight (not three) hours.[70] Another pamphlet, aimed at sailors, advised, "The prophylactic treatment, provided aboard ship, will give you some protection if taken within two hours, but it is up to you to protect yourself. There is only one SURE way to do this. Keep Away From Loose Women."[71] The pamphlets frequently provided conflicting messages about the safety and the procedure recommended. The military's lit-erature stressed that the treatment would not guarantee safety, yet the military could court-martial a soldier for contracting a venereal disease, arguing that he was in dereliction of duty.[72] General Pershing went so far as to write Surgeon General Blue, arguing, "The prophylaxis, if properly used, is so surely a protec-tion that any [case of] venereal disease arising [the soldier] must be severely punished."[73] Yet one pamphlet mentioned that venereal infections could be transmitted by innocent activities such as sharing drinking cups and utensils, demonstrating how an innocent group could be susceptible to an individuals' immoral behavior.[74]

Hygienists disagreed about the effectiveness of the procedure, although they agreed that soldiers must be taught that some treatment was better than no treatment. Reports early in the war suggested that many soldiers believed themselves doomed if they did not receive treatment within the allotted time, despite the inconsistencies of what constituted the allotted time. Others believed that syphilis was incurable, a common response to the scare tactics that dominated the popular, medical, and military literature.[75] In response, late in the war effort, the CTCA distributed a booklet entitled "Carry On." It told the story of Major Foster, a medical officer, and Corporal Harrison, a young soldier who was receiving treatment for syphilis. Foster worries over Harrison's failure to recover both physically and emotionally from his illness. Harrison tells the doctor that the disease is not what bothered him, but the stark future it promises:

> "The thing is incurable—it rots a man's bones, eats his flesh, and blinds his baby's eyes."
> "Who told you that?" demanded the Major, with a scowl.
> "Why—why, I saw it in a medical book . . ."
> "Oh," said the Major with an amused smile; "studying up on your case, eh? Well, beware, that's dangerous business. . . . You see, Harrison, medical books were written for doctors and not for patients. You surely didn't read it right. Stick to the books and the instructions the army gives you; they will tell you all you need to know."[76]

The military encouraged a soldier's better understanding of the workings of venereal diseases, provided he recognize the military hierarchy, and the medical establishment, as the source of ultimate expertise. The story reinforced both medical expertise and the importance of vigilant treatment. Foster further advises, "All I am telling you is to buck up; don't cry about the spilled milk; get well as quickly as you can; do your little stunt for Uncle Sam. Some day I expect to hear that you've made good."[77] Thus, an infected soldier, having failed to maintain his purity, could redeem himself by sticking with his treatment, performing his patriotic duty, and trusting in the medical and military establishment. Harrison not only sticks with his treatment but encourages others in the venereal hospital to do likewise, improving morale and efficiency among his fellow troops. In discussing the case later with a fellow officer, Foster muses, "If the men would only understand that they should come to us for friendly advice as well as medical advice, we could do more for them."[78] The doctors are the heroes of the story for their camaraderie with the soldiers, their training in saving lives, and their ability to replace the myths of the street with scientific fact.

The heroic doctors treated venereal disease differently based on numerous factors, but perhaps most of all on race. African American troops paradoxically faced more repressive regulations and insufficient medical attention, due in large part to racist assumptions about black sexuality. As discussed earlier, the white public and the medical establishment believed blacks to be almost universally infected with venereal diseases, particularly syphilis. VD rates among black soldiers indeed were higher than among white soldiers, but that reflected an existing bias among draft board officers rather than sexual behavior once inducted into the Army. Most draft boards assumed that black troops would serve in labor gangs, rather than in combat units, so they were less stringent on physical and health requirements for blacks. As a result, a higher percentage of blacks than whites were categorized as immediately ready for service.[79] Once in the army, they received less frequent treatments and shorter hospitalizations for the same illnesses as whites. Often contemporaries assumed this was because blacks did not suffer as much when they had venereal diseases, but the pattern had more to do with high demand for black labor than with blacks' actual health-care needs.[80]

Racism indeed affected the medical treatment received by black troops. Captain Arthur B. Spingarn, an active NAACP officer and a captain in the US Navy Sanitary Corps, wrote an article for the *Journal of Social Hygiene* in the fall of 1918, detailing some of the problems he noticed in the treatment of black soldiers. He wrote that Secretary of War Newton Baker had praised the sanitary conditions of black troops once in camp and noted that their rate of newly acquired infections "compare[d] favorably" with that of white troops.[81] What dismayed Spingarn, however, was white refusal to treat black soldiers as equals when it came to health care. Prejudice, he argued, negatively influenced the medical treatment black received. For example, black troops were required to submit to chemical prophylaxis, whether or not they claimed to have had sexual relations. Commanding officers often refused black soldiers passes to leave their bases, because they assumed the men would only get into trouble.[82] In addition, some infirmaries that served black troops did not possess sterilizers, and as a result medical attendants injected soldier after soldier with unclean syringes. This could result in possible transmission of disease from one soldier to another rather than cure or prevention. When asked about the lack of sterilization, the surgeon in charge responded, "It was useless to try to cure negroes . . . they only got infected again."[83]

Spingarn summed up his point by stating that African American troops had been abandoned by the American Plan:

> For months, in this camp, no part of the program of the War Department to safeguard the morals and health of soldiers has been put in operation as far as this group [Negroes] were concerned. . . . The only attempt to keep down the venereal rate was a rigid restriction of leaves and an enforced prophylactic treatment given to every colored soldier upon his return to camp irrespective of whether he was married or single or whether he had been exposed or not.[84]

The War Department used more coercive methods against blacks than against whites. Spingarn saw some improvement in these conditions by mid-1918, but he believed the military still had not reached equal treatment. After chiding whites for racist behavior, he appealed to whites' self-interest. He concluded by saying, "There is no such thing as white and colored disease and vice, but only disease and vice." Spingarn described how white and black soldiers both frequented black houses of prostitution and thus infection traveled across the color line. If whites continued to ignore the problem, "how long . . . before the popular notion of the prevalence of venereal disease among negroes will be the actual rate among the whites"?[85]

The VD problem in the military resulted in debate over appropriate treatment and prevention, but more fundamentally it stimulated a debate over the very nature of race, manhood, and disease. Black men and women were subject to harsh penalties and inadequate medical care. The same medical rhetoric that assumed African Americans' near-universal infection with VD in civilian circles affected the medical treatment of soldiers. Restriction and segregation, rather than education or prophylactic treatment, guided military efforts to stem black VD rates. Despite Spingarn's efforts, black soldiers' willingness to fight for the same cause did not correlate to equal treatment under the American Plan.

Sex Education

By 1918, soldiers' sex education in the military took several forms: official lectures and presentations, slide shows, distributed pamphlets, and individual counseling with personnel trained to advise men on the subject of sex. Written instruction remained the backbone of the educational efforts, although through these alternate efforts, the military targeted audiences of immigrant and illiterate soldiers who may have been unwilling or unable to read English. Historian Nina Mjagkij notes that about 16 percent of recruits were foreign born and had limited command of the English language. Up to 25 percent were considered functionally illiterate by draft examiners.[86] Therefore, the military included compulsory lectures, informal talks, and visual presentations to provide a more complete, and more compelling, education to its troops.

Medical officers made up the first line of defense against venereal disease. They had the most knowledge and were thought initially to be well situated to provide lectures and counsel the men on their behavior. The military quickly recruited "social hygiene sergeants," noncommissioned offers chosen for their ability as instructors, their discretion, and their rapport with enlisted men.[87] Officers believed that the soldiers would view sergeants as apart from the establishment, of the same class and upbringing as many of the soldiers, and as "regular men" whose advice could be trusted in much the way that an older brother's words might carry more weight than a father's or doctor's.[88]

Instructors stressed abstinence as a moral duty and the only sure way to stay healthy. The War Department believed that an efficient and patriotic soldier would choose abstinence once he understood the dangers of sexual indulgence. According to standardized syllabi provided to lecturers by the Committee on Training Camp Activities, however, the lecturers did not limit themselves to teaching abstinence. They provided the men with a much fuller sex education curriculum than most had received anywhere else. A sample syllabus included extensive lessons on anatomy, including descriptions and sometimes illustrations of the structure and function of the urethra, bladder, prostate, testicles, and penis. It then described the physiology of puberty, including physical and psychological changes, the makeup of seminal fluid, and the onset of nocturnal emissions.[89] The anatomy and physiology lessons were comprehensive, but the lecturer was instructed not to "dwell on woman's anatomy or physiology."[90] The military wanted men to understand their own health and bodies, but not women's. In addition, certain topics like masturbation were thought to provoke the wrong thoughts among audiences.

The CTCA lecture syllabi only briefly discussed the moral and spiritual implications of abstinence. The government's de-emphasis of morality is especially apparent in the official guidelines provided to hygiene lecturers. In a syllabus for use in lectures on venereal diseases, the CTCA advised speakers to discuss the prevention of venereal diseases from numerous perspectives but suggested to "make brief" the moral argument and "make . . . strong" the patriotic argument. As an example, the syllabus suggested speakers say, "The soldier or sailor disabled by venereal disease is a 'slacker.' The man who takes chances is a 'slacker' or he is 'yellow.'"[91]

The military welcomed YMCA secretaries and chaplains who wished to give further attention to moral topics to supplement the military's patriotic emphasis. Secretary V. W. Dyer of the YMCA lectured to numerous companies "on the facts and dangers in sex life. Four lectures of an hour each in one day reached a thousand men,—many of whom had never had a clear presentation of the matter in their lives."[92] These YMCA-sponsored lectures usually ended with distribution of sex education and moral training pamphlets written by M. J. Exner, the author of the Mexican prostitution report and the head of the YMCA's Sex Education Bureau. These lectures by members of voluntary associations often filled gaps in between "official" lectures. The government agreed to allow these lectures, so long as they were not compulsory, not primarily medical in nature, and "confined to the big idealistic, social, and moral issues of the day."[93] The YMCA's active program of sex education for soldiers, largely dependent on Exner's views of abstinence, character building, and the benefits of physiological knowledge, further expanded the sex education program soldiers received while in the military.

While the YMCA certainly made admirable efforts to educate the soldiers, those efforts were as segregated as the YMCA itself. The YMCA employed almost thirteen thousand white secretaries, compared to only three hundred black secretaries, for Y-huts in the United States. Y-huts housed recreational, educational, and spiritual services, serving as a home base for Y secretaries. In Europe, the nearly thirteen thousand white secretaries served with the American Expeditionary Force, with only eighty-four blacks. Besides the shortage of staff, black soldiers were often relegated to classes and lectures outside of Y-huts, often in mess halls. Those who did offer educational classes—including social hygiene lectures—to black soldiers faced even higher rates of illiteracy than among the white military population.[94] While the belief in spreading education was positive, the implementation of the policy was uneven and often constrained by racist policy.

The YMCA provided a way to combine scientific and moral education in a nondenominational way. Rather late in the war, in April 1918, the CTCA began recruiting army chaplains to work with the social hygiene division. The CTCA assumed that spiritual advisors could further influence men to pursue their physical and moral health, provided that chaplains first understood the scientific facts and the military's goal. To this end, a monthly publication entitled the *Mail Bag* was established to allow chaplains to discuss their involvement in and opinions of sex education.[95] Lieutenant William Bradley of the Sanitary Corps discussed the sex education work of chaplains in an article for the *Journal of Social Hygiene* (the publishing arm of ASHA). Connecting the sanitary problem that the military must tackle to a moral question that the churches must tackle, Lt. Bradley thought that chaplains could provide a link to more intimate conversations with the men. "Hence it is important that he himself should possess sound scientific information on the subject, so that whatever he says with regard to its purely medical aspects may harmonize with the instructions given by the medical officers and by the staff lecturers."[96] Chaplains remained divided, both on their own role in sex education and on the very necessity or usefulness of the program.

Some chaplains welcomed this opportunity to provide sex education and advice, while others shuddered at the prospect. This difference of opinion is not surprising, as chaplains represented not only various religious denominations but also various social backgrounds and generations at a time when public opinion about the necessity of sex education was evolving rapidly. The first issue of the *Mail Bag*, distributed in June 1918, included excerpts from letters on both sides of the argument. The editorial comments favored a robust sex education program for troops, with the involvement of chaplains. Chaplain J. B. Frazier of the US Navy praised the sex education program, arguing:

> It is my contention that a great deal of the suffering resulting from the subject which you treat is the result of ignorance as to the dangers of social vice. A great number of the men of the Navy come from the small towns in the country where they are not brought in contact with the dangers of a seaport town. These men need to be warned and, in my opinion, your methods will be effective.[97]

Another countered, "I am most determinedly opposed to promiscuous pamphlets and treatises on this loathsome subject." The publication then editorialized that the "loathsome subject" was "a fundamentally necessary part of every man's education."[98]

Most agreed that the religious or spiritual motive behind chastity must be used if the military's goals were to be met. "Emphasis upon the medical side is fine, but it is not enough for many fellows," wrote one chaplain who favored a stronger role in moral and sex education for chaplains.[99] Chaplain A. L. Winter of Camp Lewis, Washington, concurred: "The educational campaign is the only sane, and ultimately effective, way of dealing with the situation. This campaign can be successfully launched only as you have done it—by first presenting the medical aspects of the case."[100] Another added, "Of course all moral health must come form [sic] strengthening the will that requires an injection not of prophylaxis serum, but a pouring in of good solid moral principles."[101]

Chaplains, while confident of their ability to morally advise their troops, varied tremendously in their scientific knowledge of sex, reproduction, and venereal disease. One chaplain urged his fellows to join the crusade, "If will-power is to be properly directed, knowledge must precede it, and we cannot help believing that even the chaplain will find a few scientific facts very useful in his own attack upon moral disorders." Another wrote, "I would appreciate your [the CTCA's] literature, for here is just another way whereby a chaplain may receive scientific and needed pointers."[102] Once again, the expertise rested ultimately with the medical profession. Working in conjunction with the medical corps, chaplains made up a vital aspect of the face-to-face counseling and education that men in the American Expeditionary Force encountered, relying on interpersonal relations to complement the written word.

Ideally, medical officers, social hygiene sergeants, and YMCA secretaries ended their lectures by distributing leaflets or pamphlets for the men to review in their spare time. A printed paper could remind them of the subject matter long after the lecturer had left. The written word was the quintessential method of education in America, but some feared its use in sex education. Would the soldiers dwell too much on the pamphlets in the privacy of their barracks? Would the subject matter lead to impure thoughts?[103] The military thus prepared literature that was less frank than the material suggested for lectures, more prone to euphemism, and more focused on abstinence.

Selling abstinence to military men, after a long history of accepting sexual license, required the government to redefine masculinity.[104] Instead of displaying his sexual virility, the "new" masculine soldier would forego sex for a higher call: patriotism. The US Navy's booklet, *Live Straight If You Would Shoot Straight*, defined the new model of bravery: "Bravery in bed does not win battles. Today the greatest menace to the vitality and fighting vigor of any navy is venereal disease. . . . The escape from this danger is up to the patriotism and good sense of sailors like yourself."[105] It labeled VD as a sign of dereliction of duty or cowardice: "A sailor in the hospital with venereal disease is worse than a slacker, because he volunteers for high duty and deliberately makes himself a burden upon the navy instead of a fighting man."[106] A placard illustrated with a sketch of a fetching young woman cautioned, "If you get clap or syphilis, it's the same as if you had turned your back and run to cover."[107] Instead of linking masculinity to sexual adventure and virility, the propaganda stressed that sexual intercourse did not "make a man" of a soldier but only demonstrated his cowardice. A pamphlet aimed at sailors on shore leave advised, "If you cripple yourself by getting a disease that can easily be avoided, you are not doing your duty. . . . You must be well when you go into this fight, or you will go under. You must get the enemy, or he will get you."[108] Another pamphlet advised, "You do not need it to make a man of yourself. On the contrary, a man can not long remain a fine sample of physical vigor if he does indulge in promiscuous intercourse."[109]

In these pamphlets, the moral incentive often took a backseat to the patriotic incentive, just as medical officers concentrated on pragmatic arguments while leaving the moral rhetoric to chaplains. The *Home Reading Course for Citizen-Soldiers*, prepared by the Committee on Public Information, advised, "In addition to the moral reasons, there rests upon every soldier the especial duty of avoiding anything that may unfit him for active and effective service. This obligation in the present crisis is even greater and more urgent than in normal times."[110] The committee's emphasis on patriotism was similar to the Committee on Training Camp Activities lecture service's emphasis on patriotism and duty, leaving others to emphasize moral arguments.

One account by Fred B. Smith, a YMCA field worker in France, illustrated the effectiveness and practicality of the patriotic approach. He wrote an article stating that unofficial surveys he had conducted among YMCA members before the war and soldiers during the war demonstrated a surprising change in their moral attitudes. When asked to list the worst sins a man could commit, the prewar groups usually chose sexual immorality to top their list, followed by drunkenness, gambling, and dishonesty. For the soldiers in France, these sins fell far below cowardice and selfishness. Smith interpreted the change to mean that soldiers saw immorality as less of an immediate threat to the war effort. The true sin in sexual immorality, then, was how it endangered a soldier's fighting ability, thus risking the safety and success of his unit. Besides, a man could take precautions: "The very fact that there is a prophylactic treatment for the man who is guilty of immorality perhaps makes the offense seem less terrible to him. There is no prophylactic for cowardice, for instance."[111] Smith was careful not to take this attitude as license for promiscuity; he followed up these statements by noting the government's official stance "that these men should be warned unreservedly of danger and punished for failure to meet the regulations," which could include a court-martial, dock in pay, or worse. "If he has serious trouble [VD] as a consequence of his act, he is taken out of the army, sent back to this country—to which he has failed in duty—and, as a dishonorably discharged soldier, he may be deprived of his citizenship!"[112] Another telling of this incident hypothesized that the sins associated with "wine and women" were "a personal matter. The 'sins' that mattered were those which injured that collectivity called the army."[113] Smith believed that patriotism contributed to, and at times outweighed, the traditional moral stance against sexual promiscuity.

Relying on a favorite theme of Progressives, many pamphlets invoked efficiency as a trait of the patriotic soldier. Progressives hated to waste labor, resources, or people.[114] Like patriotism, efficiency was best achieved through informed sexual abstinence. One pamphlet advised, "Don't take a chance that risks your reputation and the strength and efficiency of your outfit."[115] Another wrote, "Neglect may mean your physical impairment and loss of efficiency."[116] The efficient, patriotic ideal soldier did not sacrifice his masculinity in order to fulfill his duty.

Propaganda borrowed from another popular image of efficient masculinity to counter the myth of sexual necessity: the athlete. Numerous publications discussed how athletes, from boxers to football players, gave up sex during training, thus saving their strength to focus their energy and concentration on the task ahead. One pamphlet advised, "Any reputable doctor will tell you that sexual intercourse is not necessary to health. Athletes from the time of the Romans to the present day cut it out during long periods of training."[117] Another booklet aimed at naval recruits wrote, "The mere fact that famous boxers and wrestlers, explorers and athletes who want their bodies to be in perfect condition for a great struggle, keep away from women during the long period of training, proves that the use of the sex organs is not necessary to health."[118] The military propaganda endeavored to challenge the notion that sexual activity proved virility by stressing an alternate, but still intensely virile, image of masculinity. Professional sports and the cult of athletics, gaining popularity in American public during the Progressive Era, provided an attractive model for soldiers to emulate.[119]

The emphasis on virile and masculine chastity may have also aimed to combat homosexuality, which was increasingly visible in training camps and port cities in the United States. Hand in hand with the threat of heterosexual prostitution, big city life and the sex-segregated world of the military opened the door for soldiers to experiment with homosexuality.[120] The literature did not address homosexuality openly, but the military was well aware of it. Historian Margot Canaday details federal immigration and military policy that inscribes heterosexuality and masculinity as traits of the soldier and citizen. Military administrators feared that the military would draw in people with same-sex attraction but also that Americans abroad would be subject to contact with "morality at variance with our own."[121] While Progressives may have hoped that military service would coerce American soldiers into more positive morality, they also feared that those same soldiers would be tempted by supposed European effeminacy or situational homosexuality. A soldier with homosexual tendencies was undesirable both as a soldier and as an American citizen, not to mention a detriment to eugenic concerns over the future of the race.

Immediately following the war, the Navy conducted a sting operation in Newport, Rhode Island, to flush out "sexual perverts" surrounding the naval base there. Before the war, the YMCA had gained a reputation as a central institution in gay male life, providing a meeting place and living quarters in which single men could congregate. Military propaganda had to balance encouraging chastity to maintain social health and discouraging any sort of feminization, which would endanger the accepted gender hierarchy. World War I was a time of competing ideas about gay identity, and the Navy investigation of homosexuality and the subsequent defense of homosocial culture in Newport in 1919 reflects that uncertainty. A reassessment in the early 1920s found the investigation immoral and accused the military of entrapment.[122] When one identified abstinence with womanhood, redefining manhood as chaste challenged the existing cultural assumptions about the divide between men and women. Abstinent and gay men both failed to live up to nineteenth century assumptions of male virility. But abstinence deserved social respect.

Military and civilian authorities agreed that sexual abstinence provided the best protection against disease and moral degeneracy. Furthermore, the military propaganda told soldiers that the benefits of sexual abstinence did not end with the armistice. It also packaged chastity as a path to upward mobility and Americanization upon return to civilian life. Those who were born into middle-class respectability would no doubt understand the duty and honor of sexual chastity because of their internalization of the supposedly national standard of conduct. Those who were not could learn it through their military experience. In a sample letter to "Son of Mine," a model patriotic mother writes, "Many of the boys who will come home with you have no mothers to write them. Some of them may think that no one cares what they do. But somebody does care. America cares."[123] This reflects a double-edged belief among Progressives about the military draft: it presented both the danger that good boys would pick up bad habits from poor and foreign-born populations and the chance to uplift that riffraff through contact with better classes. Another pamphlet appealed to the poorer soldiers' desire for economic upward mobility: "You will be a hero when you get back to the old home town. They will come out to greet you. The best jobs in politics and business will be reserved for the boys who wore the khaki. . . . *For God's sake don't spoil it.* For the sake of the Flag you fight for COME HOME CLEAN."[124] This presented the positive flip side to the threats of docked pay and courts-martial for those who contracted venereal diseases in the military. Military propaganda sold chastity during wartime and peacetime as the patriotic duty of the good soldier, as the honorable and moral thing to do, and as the healthy and responsible action.

Secretary of War Josephus Daniels included his own message in a pamphlet distributed to the Navy. He wrote, "Victory is jeopardized by the preventable diseases which destroy the fighting strength of armies and navies. It is our task to preach clean lives so as also to make democracy worth fighting for. . . . Today, as never before, American manhood must be clean and fit. America stands in need of every ounce of her strength."[125] Daniels' message was two-fold: that chastity would increase the value of the "war for democracy" and that the war created the necessity for a new vision of American masculinity. Lectures and pamphlets served the same overarching purpose with slightly different strategies. The combination of frank, anatomical lectures and aspirational pamphlets provided a curriculum that included social expectation and sexual health. The CTCA combined entertainment media with education, further expanding its curriculum.

Wholesome Recreation

In their study of venereal disease in the army, William F. Snow and Wilbur A. Sawyer looked beyond medical treatment and endorsed Fosdick's initial assessment: "It is in the soldier's playtime that he gets into trouble. Telling him what to avoid is not enough."[126] To keep the troops healthy, reformers debated the merits of shutting down saloons and bawdy houses versus chemical prophylaxis after exposure. But on one aspect of the plan all agreed: give them something else to do. The YMCA and the YWCA also attempted to arrange a more "home-like" moral atmosphere, providing wholesome recreation since the Punitive Expedition in Mexico to soldiers and to the young white women who flocked to the border in search of work.[127]

Furnishing wholesome recreation was central to the American Plan. The CTCA worked in conjunction with the YMCA, YWCA, and other religious institutions to host dances, athletic competitions, musical programs, libraries, and educational opportunities. The AEF also authorized the YMCA to operate holiday resorts for soldiers on leave. It is important to keep in mind that all of these facilities were segregated and that black soldiers rarely were able to access resources comparable to those provided to white soldiers.[128] The War Department hoped these efforts would improve white soldiers, at least, morally, physically, and intellectually.[129]

Motion pictures fast became one of the soldiers' favorite pastimes. Films were guaranteed high attendance, thus limiting the number of soldiers leaving camp for the evening. The military also selected films to strengthen the troops' moral education. Many of the films described in military catalogs provided more than mere escapism, with summaries stressing their patriotic messages and educational value. Thus, the military combined education and entertainment to complement the written or spoken word.[130] Visual displays served to attract a crowd, reinforce the literature, and reach the large segments of the population who could not read.

Before the war, sex educators took their cues from other popular health movements of the time, including traveling health exhibits and rural patent medicine shows.[131] Patent medicine hucksters often drew as much from the American dramatic tradition as from medicine, selling relief from venereal disease and other laments through showmanship and trickery more than science. They understood the importance of drawing a crowd in order to sell their product. Some salesmen created "anatomical museums," that combined the medicine show with the lure of the nickelodeon. These attractions, with a large placard reading "For Men Only" over the entrance, included a display of diseased body parts, supposedly eaten away by syphilis or gonorrhea. Disgusted and titillated viewers then met the so-called doctor who could perform a quick exam and sell a quick cure.[132] Stereopticons, slide shows, and motion pictures changed the technology through which audiences experienced a presentation.[133] Like patent medicine sellers, sex educators could use new visual media to shock their audiences with close-ups of syphilitic skin lesions or awe their audiences with the latest technology.

Mixing education and entertainment worked for both educators and entertainers, but with questionable results. Movie producers knew that sex sells, and they took advantage of that dictum as far as the state and municipal censors would allow. To bypass censors, producers would often label their films "educational," arguing that by seeing the perils of illicit sexuality, or storylines that tended to punish those who strayed from traditional sexual mores, audiences would learn restraint. Before the war, in 1913, the *New York Times* criticized early films that attracted audiences by sensationalizing current scandals. The contemporary controversy over "white slavery" sparked several exploitation films. The *Times* editorialized, "The final slide announced that its purpose was to teach a great moral lesson. What the audience saw was a representation of the sensational ways in which . . . the so-called White Slavers work. . . . Several hundred persons were turned away when the exhibition began, and a large proportion of the audience was *composed of young girls from* 16 to 18 years of age."[134] One film censor from Pennsylvania agreed. He derided theater managers who claimed they provided an educational public service but whose "lesson is mixed with a seductive story 'to get it across'; he advertises it luridly that he may draw all classes to his doors in a spirit of morbid curiosity. They do not come in a frame of mind for learning."[135] The combination of education and entertainment inspired skepticism even as it drew larger audiences.

Resistance faded during World War I when the government demanded greater publicity about venereal disease and sex education. Most in the military quickly embraced visual media as part of a necessary program of sex education. Training camps hosted slide shows and illustrated lectures to teach sexual hygiene to the troops. Physicians especially applauded the use of visual technologies to complement lectures. The *Texas State Journal of Medicine* reported in 1917 on the use of stereopticon slides to make a greater impact on their audience. Dr. H. C. Moore, chair of the Texas committee on the study of venereal diseases, wrote, "Such a lecture, attended by men or women, would be far more effective in the diminution of venereal disease than half a hundred sermons from the pulpit on personal purity." He continued, "The human mind naturally rebels at the sight of the noxious lesions which venery produces, and nothing can be more effective than a vivid illustration of them, coupled with a warning and instruction as to the methods of avoiding them."[136] That September, the *Texas State Journal of Medicine* reported on sex hygiene exhibits for recruits in Jefferson, Missouri. The Missouri State Social Hygiene Association teamed a stereopticon exhibit with a trained lecturer, noting, "The illustrations consist of diagramatic and anatomical drawings and photographs of actual cases and colored pictures designed to add to the interest of the exhibit."[137] The author's description belies the exhibit's creators intent to attract attention to the exhibit's novelty as well as to its subject matter.

The next logical step was to combine entertainment with education through the new medium of the moving picture. With military efficiency, the US Army produced the film, *Fit to Fight* in 1917, designed for screening by troops in training camps. The film opens with a lengthy segment of photographs and explanatory descriptions of venereal lesions. Then it tells the story of several recruits tempted by sin in an army training camp. Billy Hale, the hero, refuses to consort with prostitutes, therefore escaping infection and fulfilling his duty on the battlefield. Kid McCarthy, another recruit, visits a brothel but immediately reports for prophylactic treatment and thus escapes infection. The other men who visit the brothel become infected and are disqualified from foreign service. They spend the rest of the film diseased, filled with shame and regret.[138] The film combines a brief fictionalized story with the more commonly used medical exposé to tie a public health message to one of morality and patriotism.

ASHA produced and sold to the Navy an unreleased feature-length adventure film depicting sailors in a story similar to *Fit to Fight*.[139] In *Cleared for Action*, Machinist Mate Ray Eldon, the poor but patriotic hero, refuses to visit a house of prostitution with his buddies while on shore leave. His pilot, Lieutenant Mel Carter, a wealthy but sinful rogue, gets drunk, carouses with prostitutes, and fails to report for medical treatment upon his return to his ship. Both Ray and Mel fight heroically before their paths diverge upon their return home. Mel finds out he contracted a venereal disease and is unable to donate blood to save his dying fiancée. Ray, by contrast, becomes an officer and returns home to marry Mel's sister. The story ends with the caption, "WHICH LIFE WILL YOU FOLLOW?" showing Mel dejected and alone, while Ray and his wife lovingly hold their young children.[140] Both films depict a class message: abstinence leads to upward mobility for Billy Hale and Ray Eldon, while sexual indulgence ruins the wealthy Mel Carter.

Films, pamphlets, and face-to-face conversations all were to reinforce the same idea: the men of the Great War must be chaste—for their own sake, for the sake of the armed forces, and for the sake of the nation depending upon them. By using patriotism and class mobility to sell sexual abstinence, the military and the federal government turned around the image of the army from rough-and-ready sinners into one more befitting the Progressive Era's moral agenda.

In the summer of 1918, Surgeon General Rupert Blue praised the successes of the American Plan:

Now that the army is growing to millions, and every family or so has a son in it, we find it easier to arouse interest. Sources of infection are being wiped out, prostitution suppressed, alcohol prohibited, education on the subject promoted, and wholesome recreational facilities provided in camp and community. Imperfect as are our results, they represent, as far as we can tell, the best yet obtained in any part of the world.[141]

The multipronged American Plan provided a far more complete sex education program than anything available to civilians. What is more, it appeared to work. Venereal disease rates reportedly decreased significantly, although statistics vary from source to source.[142] The reformers' strategy of touting military efficiency, patriotism, and duty, combined with chemical treatments for the infected and harsh punishments for those who did not take precautions, succeeded in lowering rates of infection.

The American Plan also demonstrated how race and gender altered the meaning of sex education during wartime. Black troops received less attention from social hygiene publications, shoddy medical treatment, and fewer recreational options to lure them away from the saloon and the red light. Crackdowns on prostitution bowed to assumptions about gender and race. The military viewed nonwhite women as sexual predators who were universally infected and introduced disease to both white and black troops.

All in all, the sex education program enacted as a military necessity made great strides in presenting useful information to the soldiers. It aimed specifically at preventing and treating venereal disease, since that was considered the greatest threat to the war effort. Yet the larger picture of Progressive success hid certain failures. The military's program of sex education contradicted its own claims for success when applied to racial minorities or women. Owing to the reality of the segregated military, some soldiers benefited more than others. Some faced more coercive methods to keep them fit to fight. The military reinforced the status quo, protecting racial, gender, and class privilege.

While soldiers and sailors received the brunt of the attention from sex education reformers, they were not the only ones who needed the information. The military and its reform-minded allies worked to reach women, war industry workers, and other civilians who came into contact with soldiers. Patriotic fervor and the rhetoric of national emergency blurred the lines between soldier and civilian. Many Americans not in uniform found themselves under the watchful eye of the War Department. Social hygiene work, specifically surrounding military cantonments, gave civilians access to better sex education and gave the government an excuse to crack down on those not willing to toe the line. The fourth part of the American Plan, law enforcement, hit civilians hardest. The next chapter discusses how the war and the social hygiene movement influenced the lives of civilians.

Chapter Six

Policing Sexuality on the Home Front

In March 1918, an editorial in the *San Antonio Express* urged the city government to work with the military to clean up the city and make it a fit place for soldiers to train and people to live: "The old proverb, 'What is sauce for the goose is sauce for the gander,' is working out beautifully in those cities where the army camps are located. The army is the goose and the general public is the gander. . . . The Government has determined on certain conditions for the army camps, and these conditions are of necessity forced upon the community." The "sauce" referred to was restrictions on certain "immoral" actions, particularly drinking and prostitution. The editorial advocated prohibiting alcohol in town and ending prostitution not only for moral improvement and for the greater war effort but also for the economic advantages of complying with military orders. "The choice is clear and plain; it is a choice between the liquor business and the army business. . . . The deciding element is the dollar." The editorial also struck a moral argument: "The old idea that patriotism was a Fourth of July celebration, was a narrow view. Now we are exercising the patriotic virtues at the table, the pantry, in the bank, on the train, in moral sanitation, and in temperance reform. . . . The outcome will be seen in a greater and purer city."[1]

The editorial's multiple justifications for supporting a major vice crackdown in San Antonio demonstrate several key aspects of moral policing during World War I. It mentioned the concerns of businessmen, noting that a military presence meant a financial boom to the local economy. It placed the vice crusade in the context of a larger Progressive campaign for moral uplift. And it equated soldiers with civilians in terms of moral policing. Propagandists in the War Department used patriotism, efficiency, and national destiny to instill heightened moral codes in soldiers, and city officials did the same to civilians. San Antonio, which hosted more than seventy thousand soldiers during the war, also policed its civilians, arguing that what was good for the army was good for the community as a whole.

Did the old adage apply to an expansive sex education curriculum? The American Social Hygiene Association and the Commission on Training Camp

Activities advocated sex education for civilians, but strategies accepted for use by the Army were not always considered good for private citizens. Yet, in many areas surrounding training camps and military bases, the line between civilian and military was blurred. The fervor with which the military embraced sex education and the American Plan spilled over onto the home front, suggesting that the government saw little difference between soldiers and civilians in facilitating an efficient and patriotic war effort. Government advertising to save food and buy bonds encouraged those not serving abroad, such as women and industrial workers, to take part in the war effort. Propaganda also encouraged citizens back home to live straight, avoid VD, and serve their nation as moral guardians of the American way.

The government perceived private citizens as a possible threat to the war effort, which justified the military's expansion into civilian regulation. By 1918, the military had determined that most soldiers did not become infected with venereal diseases while in the Army but came to the Army already infected. Studies consistently attributed five-sixths of VD infections to civilian life, and only one-sixth infections that occurred while under the watchful eye of the military.[2] Thus, to protect soldiers, the problem must be stopped at the root: civilian life. Women represented the largest perceived threat to the moral side of the war effort. Yet women's image in the war effort was multifaceted. They were celebrated as mothers, workers, and symbols of American purity. Conversely, they could endanger men's fighting capacity through their sexual aggression and disease. Representations of women in the wartime sex education crusade often reduced them to either good girls (mothers, sisters, and sweethearts), who served as the motivation to keep soldiers moral, or bad girls (prostitutes, "charity girls,"[3] or women unlucky enough to be in the wrong place at the wrong time). Military and civilian authorities labeled deviant girls a "menace" to soldiers and the war effort. Reformers saw sex education and the policing of sexuality as part of the war effort. They aimed to guide people to the ideals of the chaste, patriotic life and to punish and coerce those who strayed. World War I exacerbated divisions among women based on class and racial identity. The modest gains made by white middle-class women through collaboration with antivice crusades were achieved to the detriment of younger, poorer, more marginalized women.

This chapter analyzes sex education efforts aimed at civilian women during World War I. The movement was national, but the federal government and its allies focused their efforts where they were most concerned about results: in the proximity of soldiers. Cities like San Antonio, Texas, were prime targets of vice control because of large populations of soldiers, multiracial communities, and the presence of female detention homes.

The military and civilian antivice campaign during World War I demonstrates three important aspects of the Progressive sexual agenda. First, gender played a crucial role in the antivice activism. Despite not having the vote, women drew on their maternal, pure reputations to carve a niche for themselves as political activists, social workers, and police officers. Therefore, activists advocated rehabilitation or education as well as punishment. Second, the antivice campaign clearly delineated differences among women of different classes and ethnic identities. Middle-class white reformers used the antivice campaign as a path to greater political power, but, in so doing, they denied the same rights and privileges to working class and nonwhite women. Finally, women who had previously been viewed as the victims of prostitution now were labeled (and treated) as powerful and dangerous forces in their own right. Some women's "khaki fever" (the appeal of a man in uniform) and unbridled sexuality was a threat to the health of soldiers, the war effort, and the very standards of American society.

Wartime Sex Education for Girls

Prior to the war, ASHA advocates had constructed arguments favoring limited sex education programs for women and girls. Within the white middle-class population, sex education was viewed more as a tool for protecting girls from male sexual exploitation than for fostering self-awareness. Class and racial assumptions complicated reformers' image of girlhood and sexual maturity, because they assumed white middle-class girls had a different, and purer, sexual experience than other girls. Evidence of a girl's sexual precocity or aggressiveness lowered her class and racial status and placed her outside the realm of chivalrous protection.

ASHA continued its involvement in girls' protective work, as well as the educational measures that accompanied it. In March 1918, the *Social Hygiene Bulletin* warned of the dangers of "the lure of the uniform" and praised the work of the War Department's Committee on Protective Work for Girls. ASHA and the CTCA developed educational programs aimed at girls and their mothers. In Atlanta, Georgia, the committee went so far as to open a free ward and dispensary for the treatment of "delinquent" girls.[4] Efforts to improve girls' understanding of sexuality and its dangers expanded tremendously because of the military emergency.

The CTCA's Section on Women's Work distributed pamphlets to mothers and daughters similar to those dispensed to soldiers. The pamphlets' purpose was to teach women appropriate sex education lessons while promoting the values considered necessary to help the war effort. *Mothers of America*, by Dr. Mabel S. Ulrich, was a pamphlet released by the CTCA specifically for "members and other adult women." The CTCA wanted to protect parental prerogative and insert an intermediary between the government and the girls. Perhaps because it was not expected to go directly to girls, *Mothers of America* provided direct and detailed lessons in reproduction, anatomy, and sexual hygiene.[5]

Mothers of America justified breaking the conspiracy of silence just as the literature aimed at soldiers did. The pamphlet publicized VD statistics and warned of the deleterious effects on military efficiency. "In the past, we have had the excuse, such as it was, of ignorance. To-day the war has brought us face to face, not with theories, but with unescapable [*sic*] facts and figures. The time for silence and drifting is over. The war has forced the issue of sex education." First, the pamphlet cautioned mothers about the dangers of khaki fever. "Many girls . . . have lost their heads over uniforms. They [military officials] will tell you that their problems include by no means only the girls who are in industry, but girls in the automobile class as well, and young girls often in the seventh and eighth grades at school." The "automobile class" signified those wealthy enough to own automobiles, the middle and upper classes. The warning refuted the basic assumptions held by many reformers: that only working-class girls and adult women had the potential to be sexually aggressive.[6] Ulrich urged middle-class women to take seriously the sexual threat in their own social circles.

Ulrich placed the responsibility directly on mothers to educate their daughters. She instructed mothers how to field questions by curious children, including frank questions about reproduction. Ulrich suggested a mother explain not just how mothers carry children but how fathers fertilize eggs: "Here the mother should make it perfectly clear that the penis is meant."[7] The pamphlet encouraged mothers to educate girls about menstruation before it occurs and explain that it is not a disease. Ulrich agreed with women physicians and reformers who challenged medical assumptions that female sexual development was debilitating or pathological.

Ulrich's method of appealing to mothers or girls' protective workers was in keeping with the general strategy adopted by the Section on Women's Work. The section suggested a three-pronged approach, including education first for mothers, then for girls' club leaders, and finally for the girls themselves. To that end, the section established suggested programs for women's clubs including lectures, discussion groups, and visual presentations.[8]

Mrs. Rose Woodallen Chapman, author of numerous education publications, also published sex education pamphlets for the Commission on Training Camp Activities. She connected sexual restraint to patriotism, accusing promiscuous girls of "playing the Kaiser's game." In *The Nation's Call to Young Women*, Chapman called sexually active men and women the enemy. Just as a man was accused of being a slacker if he exposed himself to VD, a girl who slept with soldiers, or even sexually excited them, was a "traitor."[9] Chapman stressed that it was part of a girl's duty to the war effort to resist sexual temptation, for her own sake, the sake of the soldiers, and for the future of the race. Her pamphlet briefly described the consequences of syphilis and gonorrhea, and while not as explicit as Ulrich, Chapman assumed that knowledge of diseases and the ways they are spread was vital to stemming the epidemic.

Chapman's second pamphlet, *Your Country Needs You*, was rife with eugenic rhetoric, noting the dangerous consequences of a war that had the potential of killing off the finest citizens. "You will be the next generation of parents. The responsibility for future generations rests on your shoulders." She then described the anatomy of the female reproductive system and the process of menstruation. "Now you can begin to see why you are expected to take such extra good care of yourself at each menstrual period." The focus of sex education was not physical pleasure but fulfillment through motherhood and its contribution to the race. For that reason, both premarital sexual activity and masturbation were characterized as physically and psychologically harmful.[10] Furthermore, Chapman assumed that girls would not understand the nature of their sexual impulses. She relied to a degree on the doctrine of passionlessness, assuming that proper women found physical fulfillment not in the sex act but in maternity: "These are, really, expressions of the wonderful instinct which is leading you on gradually to the time when, fully developed physically, mentally, and morally, you will be prepared to marry and to call other human beings into existence. Until that time arrives you have no right to use your creative powers, nor should you allow the racial impulses or passions to be stirred within you." Chapman expressed mixed feelings regarding the concept of "race," attributing both the positive eugenic connotation of contributing to the perpetuation of the "race" and the dangerous side of "racial impulses." Chapman's use of the word "race" conflated ideas of the human race and more specific, ethnically charged stereotypes.[11] Sexuality was connected to "racial" impulses both in the human race and within specific racial groups. Chapman implied that sexual excitement was a racial stain on white girlhood, calling into question their purity and their whiteness.

Many of the pamphlets emphasized women's power to change the world through their influence over men. One argued:

> Women can stop prostitution by taking a definite stand in this matter. . . . Never before in the history of any country has there been such an opportunity for social progress, for social justice, for individual ideals as this which faces our country at this time; never before have the women and girls of any country had such an opportunity to make their convictions so felt and their ideals count for so much.[12]

This propaganda related women's power to remaking the world, but not through a political voice. Theirs was the maternalist, not feminist, influence as mothers, wives, and moral protectors. Progressives often utilized this strategy to circumvent male and female resistance to equal-rights feminism. Maternalists and feminists made different arguments to justify women's rights, including suffrage. Maternalists highlighted the supposed differences between the sexes, arguing that women's superior moral stature, incorruptibility, and nurturing instincts would make them ideal political citizens.[13]

In spite of maternalist and feminist support of sex education, there was a backlash against the rapid change in the "conspiracy of silence" and the interaction of the sexes. One pamphlet reflected a minority view within the YWCA about the American Plan. The author of *Why Our Women Are Frightened* was aghast at the actions the YWCA took to help the war effort. The pamphlet criticized the government's "immoral arrangements . . . for the entertainment and gratification of these beastly men [soldiers]." Agreeing with Chapman, the pamphlet feared that "modern dancing" and the enticing new styles girls wore to dances would lead soldiers "down rather than upwards." It blamed women with painted faces, scanty clothing, and careless posture for the problem of prostitution and venereal disease. Echoing Chapman's analysis that even chaste girls' behavior could incite a man to seek out a prostitute, the pamphlet urged a return to evangelism rather than entertainment.

That pamphlet did not represent the affirmed YMCA or YWCA position. Both Y groups advocated the American Plan and worked in conjunction with the CTCA to provide wholesome recreation and dances for enlisted men. It was a critique from within the Y organizations that challenged the union of Christian principles and the American Plan. The pamphlet warned Y girls:

> If you continue in this line of conduct, you will have to be held responsible for the blood of these young men who come under your influence, for the blood of the young women who may fall in consequence, and before your Maker you will have to account for the opportunities which you have had and which you have neglected to make use of in bringing these young men and women to the true knowledge of Him.[14]

This memorandum, not published by the Y's Association Press, took a more dismal view of the American Plan, and indeed the future of American society, than most Y literature. It viewed sex education and light recreation as detrimental both to health and to men's and women's souls. This dissent from within the Y indicates that the military and its allied reformers had failed to gain universal approval for their involvement in preventing venereal diseases.

Some of the tactics and strategies the government used to keep soldiers safe from venereal disease changed significantly when applied to women. For example, while the propaganda for soldiers stressed the benefit of upward class mobility through pure and patriotic duty, the movie *The End of the Road*, produced for civilian women, warned against class aspirations. Written by Katherine Bement Davis of the CTCA and released for civilian audiences in 1918, the film followed a formula similar to *Fit to Fight* but focused on women instead of men. The two main characters, Mary Lee and Vera Lynch, are shaped by their mothers' teachings. The audience first meets Mary, who discovers a nest of eggs while out walking with her mother, a reference to nature study as the safest method of teaching girls about sex and reproduction. The film summary describes Mary's mother "taking [Mary] into her arms, simply and lovingly she tells her the story of her own entrance in to the world."

As a contrast, Mary's friend Vera is taught by her mother that asking about the origins of life was "naughty; good little girls never ask such questions." When caught "spooning" with a fellow, Vera's mother chastises her not for her actions but for her companion's poor economic prospects. She advises Vera to "put her hair up and try to meet older men," violating a major tenet of the sex education movement, which discouraged precocity in adolescents. Vera's mother instills in her daughter the importance of marrying well to improve her class status. As a result, in the film, Vera falls prey to a man and is seduced, jeopardizing her future and her health.[15] The film cautioned women that aspirations for "the finer things," combined with the influence of a bad mother, could lead them sexually astray.[16] Vera's boyfriend refuses to marry her after they begin living together. He deserts her, and Vera turns to Mary for help, who urges her to see a doctor. Vera, of course, has contracted syphilis. Mirroring a similar scene in *Fit to Fight*, the victim tours a medical facility to see the ravages of venereal disease, presented to the audience as well through the use of clinical photography. Vera agrees to undergo treatment and is saved.

As a contrast to Vera's sad tale, Mary represents the ideal of informed chastity. Thanks to her mother's training, Mary's moral idealism inspires her to become a nurse, where she eventually meets and marries a successful surgeon. Hence, Mary achieves the upward mobility Vera desired by staying pure. Mary and her fiancée both proclaim the benefits of sex education. The doctor counsels, "If young men could only know . . . what suffering their sowing of wild oats can mean to their wives." Mary agrees, adding, "And if girls could only know the consequences . . . they'd try to help them resist temptation." When the United States enters the war, Mary and her husband work at an Army hospital at a cantonment, where Mary assists more working-class girls who have followed the soldiers in hopes of a good time.[17]

Two things set *The End of the Road* apart from its precursors. First, it was aimed at civilian audiences, primarily women. Second, it presented women as sexual actors who made choices about their own lives. Vera is not forced by white slavers or economic necessity into moral laxity; rather, it is her early lack of sex education and her own quest for romance, adventure, and wealth that doom her. Mary, uniting patriotic impulses with sexual chastity, succeeds everywhere that Vera fails. Like the male star of *Fit to Fight*, she lives happily ever after.

Because it was created for civilian, mixed-gender audiences, the film sparked resistance immediately. The National Catholic War Council, which had built an uneasy coalition with the CTCA during the war, protested loudly after the Armistice. The council launched an all-out campaign against social hygiene films, claiming that "the entire program of the Social Hygiene section of the commission is damnable."[18] Other religious, moral, and purity organizations followed suit, questioning the necessity of "emergency" measures once the war had ended. Postwar protesters condemned sex education films on two points: the content of the films and the content of the audiences. One study concluded, "The women expressed the opinion that the film might be shown to young girls without harm. . . . In contrast to this, the majority of the men objected to the showing of the film to women."[19] Men seemed to worry more about women's supposed delicacy than the women themselves did. In the summer of 1919, the US Interdepartmental Social Hygiene Board granted psychologists Karl S. Lashley and John B. Watson $6,600 to investigate the psychological effects these films had on the civilian public.[20] Lashley and Watson arranged for viewings of the films *Fit to Win* (the civilian version of *Fit to Fight*, which portrayed Billy returning home to civilian life) and *The End of the Road* by various audiences. One showing in a small town in Pennsylvania raised particular concerns, because it included an audience "of about equal numbers of both sexes. Fully half were boys and girls below the age of seventeen."[21] It was at this showing that the young boys and girls discussed the film after leaving the theater, and "innuendo prevailed in their talk. However, investigations in the town failed to reveal that there had been any bad after-effects of this, or that parents felt that any serious problem had arisen." Their research indicated that the films did not incite immoral or impure thoughts among those who watched them, but the psychologists still recommended screenings to gender-segregated audiences to avoid any further relaxation of moral behavior.[22]

Lashley and Watson also discussed the racial makeup of audiences for the films. They held four screenings in a small town in Maryland, to accommodate a separate showing each for white men, white women, black men, and black women.[23] Afterward, Lashley and Watson theorized that the films' emotionalism and sense of drama appealed even more to African American audiences than to white audiences. "Not only were the Negroes more interested and enthusiastic than the whites in their immediate response to the picture, but later inquiries showed that a much larger per cent had been influenced to seek medical advice."[24] This conclusion draws upon two stereotypes many whites held at the time: that African Americans had high rates of venereal diseases and that their emotionalism outweighed logic. Thus, Lashley and Watson approved of using sensationalistic methods to reach African American audiences but cautioned against such tactics when addressing white or "educated" audiences.

For all audiences, Lashley and Watson concluded that the danger in combining an entertaining love story with the educational message far outweighed the benefit it might have in drawing a larger audience or keeping that audience's attention. Film censor Ellis Paxson Oberholtzer agreed. He posited that *Fit to Fight / Fit to Win* and *The End of the Road* might have had their place in training camps but were ill suited to a civilian audience. He quoted one sympathetic anonymous reviewer who remarked, "The dominant feeling with which one comes away from such films is that, if one cannot be 'good' one should be 'careful.'" Oberholtzer accused the films of removing the moral idealism Progressives espoused, leaving only "a crude appeal to the emotions."[25] The National Catholic War Council agreed, writing, "Out of fear simply of physically evil consequences nothing can come when the danger of such consequences are removed. Purity is not simply abstinence from sexual indulgence: purity is the moral life of the soul."[26]

Even sex education advocates were troubled by the use of movies to educate audiences. They admitted that the government films had some redeeming qualities, but Oberholtzer saw the real threat in films that emulated this education-through-sensational-entertainment model. This is not to say that he opposed sex education; like many Progressives, he saw it as a good idea ill suited to the theater:

> The good which can accrue from instructing the young about such a topic under proper circumstances I would not underrate. But to cry sex disease from high places with a view to leading the population for a price into a theatre—men, women and children, adolescent boys and adolescent girls, to sit to music, side by side, while the subject is developed . . . through the medium of a wishy-washy love story, perhaps to be followed or preceded, as the case may be, by a "slap-stick" comedy, is in my judgment contrary to public policy.[27]

Once again, the author stressed the dangers not just of the subject matter but of the audience makeup and setting. He criticized movie houses in which serious subjects were combined with lighter fare and in which young boys and girls could giggle together over titillating suggestions and perhaps then make some of their own.

Sex education advocates wished to make good use of visual media to attract attention to their subject matter or to "get it across," but at heart they did not want to stir up the wrong kind of interest in their subject matter. Mixing serious topics with sensationalism drew a bigger crowd, but it also invited harsher criticism from censors, medical professionals, and reformers. Without the context of national emergency during World War I, sex education films no longer seemed worth the risk. When sexual dalliance and venereal disease threatened the military's strength or efficiency, the government willingly intervened to teach large audiences through the use of film. Outside of the training camps, conversely, social hygiene programs using new media found themselves with more enemies than allies.[28] Some conservatives reluctantly went along with sex education programs for soldiers but refused to budge when the matter became one for civilians, especially women. Many reformers still categorized women's sexual behavior as deviant and advised repression, punishment, and detention rather than education.

Punishing Female Sexuality

At least a decade before the war, physicians and reformers began to acknowledge that not all girls were "passionless."[29] The emerging field of psychiatry included discourse and diagnosis of the female hypersexual, although class and racial hierarchies still tended to label those outside of the white middle class as hypersexual. It was wage-earning girls who were most often so classified. In fact, what was abnormal among white adolescent girls was expected among blacks, as medical experts used racialized notions of sexuality to categorize all blacks as naturally immoral.[30]

During wartime, female hypersexuality took on new and dangerous meanings. Parents, reformers, and the military police decried the effects of khaki fever. For some adolescent girls and young women, patriotism did not mean adhering to the War Department's standards of chastity. Rather, they apparently saw it as their patriotic duty to be sexually available to the soldiers.[31]

Appalled by girls' behaviors around the training camps, CTCA head Raymond Fosdick established a Committee on Protective Work for Girls in September of 1917. The goal of girls' protective work was not just to save girls from exploitative situations, but also to steer them into more appropriate gender and sexual roles. The problem of khaki fever indicated the public's recognition that female sexuality was not always passive, even among white, middle-class, respectable girls. Uncontrolled female sexuality threatened the military through corruption of the troops. Fosdick's response to khaki fever demonstrated a fear of "charity girls" who were diseased and promiscuous, even if they were not technically prostitutes. Across the nation, courtrooms and public opinion labeled women who entered into casual sexual relationships as prostitutes whether or not they traded money for sex.

Several women's rights activists challenged the government's American Plan, noting that the plan provided venereal disease treatment for men, while women often were detained or punished rather than treated and set free. The plan left women vulnerable while men's sins were forgiven in the interest of a quick cure. Women had previously expressed dissatisfaction with the sexual double standard, as formalized by Britain's Contagious Disease Acts of the 1860. In a 1910 nursing textbook, Lavinia Dock voiced her disenchantment with Britain's policies against contagious disease. She argued, "Punishment[s] meted out to the women were chiefly hypocritical or vindictive, not in the least preventive."[32] These arguments, chiefly criticizing police-sponsored or regulated prostitution, also applied to the way in which the detention and punishment of prostitutes adversely affected both women's rights and the cause of social health. She disapproved of the British system, which allowed men medical treatment and continued access to women but punished women for acquiring venereal diseases. Her arguments echoed those made by ASHA pioneer Prince Morrow, who theorized in 1901 that regulated prostitution discriminated against women. Notably, Morrow and Dock both feared that male police officers could abuse their power over economically, politically, and legally vulnerable women.[33]

Extrapolating from Dock's work, Edith Houghton Hooker best articulated the feminist critique of the American Plan. Hooker, who studied medicine at Johns Hopkins University before pursuing a career in social work, was dedicated to both sex education and woman suffrage, and she saw the plan's implementation destroying women's health as well as their political and legal power. Hooker picked apart the Navy's arguments supporting medical prophylaxis. She argued that the 99.6 percent success rate was false, especially considering the challenges soldiers faced getting treatment in time.[34] Foremost, she argued that the medical treatment policy the military adopted was merely a new form of regulated prostitution. Men received treatment; women received detention. For example, in 1919 in Los Angeles, California, more than 96 percent of women arrested and diagnosed with VD were quarantined, compared to only 49 percent of arrested men. Men had the opportunity to leave if they promised to seek treatment, a right denied women.[35] Similarly, historian Kimberly Jensen has found that in Portland, Oregon, women were detained while men received treatment and were released.[36] The double standard, Hooker complained, was unchallenged: "A man cannot have promiscuous intercourse alone. It is therefore obviously illogical and ethically unsound for the government to propose a system of repression directed at one sex alone."[37]

Hooker turned the patriotic argument on its head, stating that "every prostitute is a potential worker and mother," reaffirming the importance of all women to the war effort and the nation's future.[38] Women's contributions were lauded in the propaganda but not considered equal to men's. In addition, their subordinate status, both economically and politically, made them more vulnerable to state intervention in their lives. Gender played a significant role: women, especially young and socially or economically marginalized women, lacked the political standing that men possessed when confronting the power of the state, especially as the state expanded its power during the war.

It is not surprising that wartime policies pitted government against women's rights. Federal and local authorities remained skeptical of many women's organizations that had been closely tied to the peace movement. Women-led peace organizations, such as Jane Addams's Women's International League for Peace and Freedom, were shunted to the side by moderate women who embraced preparedness campaigns to demonstrate their commitment, and contribution, to the war effort.[39] The moderate suffrage movement, represented by the National American Woman Suffrage Association, distanced itself from more radical, feminist organizations such as the National Woman's Party and the National Peace Party. Some women advocated suffrage as a force for moderation, expediency, and the maintenance of nativist white supremacy.[40] During World War I, women's war work was linked closely with the question of woman suffrage; if men demonstrated their citizenship through service in the armed forces, women demonstrated their citizenship through their own contributions to the war effort. President Wilson eventually supported suffrage as an expedient measure to ensure women's continued support of the war.[41]

Dramatic events such as the National Woman's Party picketing the White House and the subsequent hunger strike of female prisoners reinforced the link between feminism and subversion for many moderate and conservative politicians.[42] Many antifeminists attributed the threat to the patriarchal family to sexual radicalism intertwined with political radicalism, using figures like Emma Goldman as their example. Defending the safety and sanctity of motherhood was one of America's justifications for the war, and indeed it justified the repression of women who somehow fell outside the sexual roles assigned to them. Women's subversion of the war effort was seen as part of the nation's larger problems of sexual degeneracy and gender perversion.[43] The developing acceptance of women's political and sexual selves caused discomfort among many—and panic among a few. With that in mind, it is not surprising that repression against those who challenged the sexual status quo, just as with political radicals, increased during the war years.

Detention homes for wayward girls did not originate during World War I, but wartime mass arrests overwhelmed existing detention facilities. Historian Jennifer Koslow describes the repression of the war era as a change in scale, not scope. The war provided the catalyst the federal government and local authorities needed to develop the infrastructure and demand the state authority necessary to expand their programs exponentially.[44] A government manual for social hygiene officers noted that the establishment of wartime detention homes began in April 1918: "It developed out of the efforts made to affect a law-enforcement program suppressing vice and liquor about the military training camps." The manual argued that these detention homes provided a better place than prison for girls to go "while awaiting trial, to be studied and treated medically." Only the "hardened cases" went directly to jail.[45]

Those orchestrating the crackdown believed that immoral women controlled or instigated sexual activity. This illustrates a shift in the public understanding of prostitution, viewed predominantly a crime of victimized girls (white slavery) before World War I, to a crime of dangerous "autonomous females." This was a double-edged sword, which historian Brian Donovan notes provided "a more realistic and enlightened image of womanhood [and] a rationale for gender discrimination."[46] By categorizing prostitution as a threat to national security, the federal government justified massive prosecution of women "reasonably suspected" of carrying venereal diseases. The military arrested and detained more than fifteen thousand women on suspicion of prostitution or disease, holding them without trial for an average of ten weeks. Only one-third were ever charged with prostitution while the rest were merely labeled promiscuous. Occupants of the

girls' reformatories often stayed longer than a year, which meant intern-
ment long after the war had ended.[47]

The broad nature of the "reasonable" suspicion of prostitution played into
class and racial assumptions about women's sexuality. Most of the detained
were identified as working class.[48] Other historians have pointed out that
efforts to "save" or "protect" delinquent girls often crossed class lines, with
middle-class women hoping to help working-class girls. Yet their efforts rarely
crossed racial boundaries; white women activists rarely worked to assist African
American or Mexican American women.[49]

Mrs. Martha P. Falconer, superintendent of a detention home for girls,
noted, "Everywhere there is forced upon us a growing realization of the menace of the immoral colored girls and women, and the difficulties in many of
the states of arousing public sentiment to make provision for their care." Falconer argued that while the military and civilian authorities were handling the
relatively minor problem of delinquent white girls, the larger problem of delinquent nonwhite girls was neglected because of institutional segregation and
apathy of white reformers. Falconer pleaded for more action, pointing out that
"the problem of the immoral colored girls and women directly affects [whites]
and is theirs to face as much as it is for the colored themselves."[50] Notwith-
standing Falconer's plea, many reformers treated the problem of black female
sexual delinquency as a hopeless cause or a chronic condition, one unlikely to
be solved and unworthy of intense effort. The only true solution was to keep
dangerous women away from soldiers.

Detention homes were established to do more than just protect soldiers
from infected women. The hope was that detention could reform and improve
inmates through educational and vocational training. Thomas A. Storey's 1922
report on the creation of detention homes across the nation stipulated the
importance of making them rehabilitation centers or "suitable places for long-
term commitment for women and girls." Specifically, he complained that there
were too few homes for African American women and girls in the South.[51] The
government specified that black and white girls would be treated with "equal
consideration wherever this might be possible," but the results did not live up
to the promise. Facilities for African Americans received less adequate funding
and were located in poorer buildings, if they existed at all. Usually, the lack of
facilities simply meant that black women and girls more often ended up in jail
rather than a detention home.[52]

Storey's coauthor, Mary Macey Dietzler, expressed concern that some of
the girls detained were so uncontrollable that they would resort to homosexual behavior while in custody. Her informants told her that this problem was
"largely among the colored girls."[53] The fear of homosexuality reflected racial
fears across the country in both segregated and nonsegregated areas. Historian
Cheryl Hicks, studying incarcerated women in New York, notes that court and
prison officials expressed fear that interracial same-sex relationships would

develop among inmates in nonsegregated prisons. Officials assumed that black women, who lacked recognition of their femininity, would play the male role and white women the female role in mimicry of heterosexuality. This assumption also labeled black women as sexually deviant, while it maintained the supposed heterosexuality of white women who sought relations with "masculine" black women.[54] Segregated homes, where possible, were the answer to prevent the danger of interracial liaisons, sexual or otherwise.

Ideally, the detention homes and reformatories provided schooling along with medical treatment to its inmates. Supervisors distributed educational materials and occasionally lectured or showed motion pictures. In homes for African American girls, however, these amenities were often left out. Inmates of the Dorcas Home for Colored Girls, in Houston, Texas, received limited "prevocational" training in cooking and domestic service, but they did not receive any education, outdoor recreation, or books. "Stories are told of severe corporal punishment under a former superintendent who was discharged, happily, as soon as her board heard of her conduct."[55] Conditions at the Dorcas Home emulated a prison more than a rehabilitation facility, and Dietzler's report confirmed this when discussing how many inmates were required to be retested for venereal disease after release:

> When the time was up they were all found to be reinfected, pointing to carelessness in the home and too great freedom of movement. The colored superintendent at that time was lax and the girls came and went without much restriction. This situation was the basis of a recommendation made by the director of the Houston Foundation that government assistance be discontinued, and that the colored population be urged to increase its efforts to supplement the city and county appropriation for maintenance.[56]

Resistance to providing rehabilitation to African American girls resulted both from the lack of resources and from a lack of interest.

The establishment of detention homes and reformatories aimed to provide an alternative to jail for women and girls considered a threat to the soldiers or the military effort. These included women suspected of engaging in prostitution or suspected of carrying venereal disease, but neither of these charges needed to be proven to land a woman in state custody. The suspension of habeas corpus and other civil rights for women marked a low point in the wartime effort to control sexuality. Reformers framed their work as beneficial rather than threatening. They argued that they were protecting soldiers, civilians, families, the war effort, and the girls themselves. The girls received medical treatment, housing, and education or vocational training while in custody. Their educational program often included a vigorous sex education program similar to that given to soldiers in training camps. At heart, however, detention demonstrated the restrictions placed on citizens based on gender and race assumptions. The crime was not any suspected sexual activity, but female, often black or Mexican American, suspected sexual activity. Reformers believed they could train girls to change their wayward lives. In practice, detention served to remove the girls from their proximity to soldiers and took away their freedom; Maude Miner, the director of the War Department's Committee for the Protection of Women and Girls, resigned over the contradictions she saw between protecting and punishing girls.[57] The focus on rehabilitation was reserved for whites only, and limited even for them.

The idea that prostitution sprang from a lack of education, and thus that prostitutes could be rehabilitated, emerged before the war. Hugh Cabot, a participant in the Fourth International Congress on School Hygiene, stated in 1913, "The prostitute is a result, not a cause. A demand has created a supply. Can it be that this demand is a result of our lack of teaching?" He blamed prostitution not on a lack of female moral control or on economic desperation but on the dual problems of lack of education and the male demand for sex. Since Cabot blamed men both for soliciting sex and for failing to provide women with education, he logically concluded that men should bear the brunt of punishment for the crime. He recognized, however, that even equal punishment of men would result in social outrage. "If we arrest and fine these women for soliciting, it is our clear duty to arrest, fine or imprison her male companion for soliciting or employing her. Does anyone in his senses believe that an attempt to enforce such a regulation would end in anything but riot?"[58] By 1917, the double standard that Cabot criticized had reached its apogee in the wartime detention of women.

Sex and the Southern City: Cleaning Up Vice in San Antonio

"San Antonio is the army center of the United States. We have 70,000 soldiers here—one cantonment, an army post, aviation fields, officers' schools, rifle ranges, and other camps."[59] The municipal and economic leaders of San Antonio, Texas, understood the benefits of keeping a military base in the area. An article in the *San Antonio Express* remarked, "War, the greatest ill wind creation knows, has blown good to the big City of Texas, good in measureless fashion."[60] San Antonio offered a warm climate, ample railroad connections, and existing military installations remaining from the Punitive Expedition in Mexico. With good reason, San Antonio expected to be a major base for the training and stationing of troops. Military and civilian officials worried that the city's historical toleration of vice, its racially diverse population, and its relative proximity to Mexico detracted from the city's assets.

After the war, however, social hygiene advocates described San Antonio as a major success story, in direct contrast to another Texas city, El Paso. El Paso illustrated the dangers of refusing to join in the military's fight against venereal disease and prostitution. In the spring of 1917, the federal government designated both San Antonio and El Paso supply depots for the Southern Department. The *Social Hygiene Bulletin* warned that southwestern cities like San Antonio and especially El Paso had a "serious obstacle" in their "presence of Mexican and Indian laborers who are unintelligent in these matters [vice] and impatient of any regulative measures."[61] It was concern over liquor and women that made one city a military success story, the other a noted failure.[62]

San Antonio newspapers extolled the virtues and enumerated the profits to be had by a military presence. To receive these benefits, San Antonio had to tackle a major perceived problem: sex. According to northeastern stereotypes, southerners and westerners tolerated the presence of prostitution and liquor. San Antonio could be identified as both southern and western, a booming frontier town with a Mexican and Confederate heritage. The War Department feared that the city's lax enforcement of vice regulations would contribute to dangerous levels of venereal disease and disorderly conduct. In response, national organizations like ASHA, as well as local San Antonio women's clubs, took it upon themselves to clean up the city and make it a model for other cantonment towns. Their success required intense pressure on the local municipal authorities and police force, and a crackdown on the civil rights of women, especially racial minorities. Progressive reformers targeted groups based on race, gender, and relative power, demonstrating the dangerous side effect of social engineering in times of war.

San Antonio stood to benefit immensely from the military presence. The early boomtown witnessed an even bigger boom as training camps and airfields moved into the surrounding area. The results were extraordinary. "San Antonio has never experienced such prosperity as she is experiencing today," said Mayor Sam C. Bell in October of 1917. The *San Antonio Express* noted that both the city and the surrounding rural community benefited from the influx of government money, especially in real estate.[63] The town boasted 133,000 permanent residents, who were joined by the beginning of 1918 by about 80,000 soldiers, 25,000 family members of servicemen, and 20,000 other temporary visitors.[64] An editorial mentioned the benefits to the city government of such cooperation between municipality and military: "In the midst of a [drought]-stricken country we have been prosperous because of the war conditions."[65] The war promised economic security and prosperity to a region that had suffered its share of economic hardships.

In January 1918, the federal government began to publicly question San Antonio's effectiveness at cleaning up its vice districts. Major Bascom Johnson, personal representative of Secretary Baker, expressed concern that the town had not fulfilled its promise to eradicate prostitution and saloons in the areas surrounding the training camps. With the local economy depending on the influx of thousands of soldiers, Johnson issued a veiled threat: the War Department could punish the city economically by removing the troops. Such a move would also damage the city's image and public relations. In response, Reverend S. J. Porter preached at the First Baptist Church that San Antonio should demonstrate its patriotism to the entire world by its actions in the antivice crusade.[66] Major Bascom Johnson concurred, adding, "If you don't do this San Antonio will be smeared to the country as a city which did not rise to its duty; that it permitted vice conditions to thrive; that thousands of improper women thronged your streets and that as a result a high disease rate spread among the soldiers stationed here, rendering them unfit for service for which the country so urgently needs them."[67] Matters intensified a few days later, when Johnson informed the city that the War Department "will take no more promises." He openly charged the city and county officials with dereliction in their duty to enforce antivice laws. "We hope the citizens and officials of San Antonio will take such action as will make unnecessary any drastic action by the War Department relating to the concentration of troops here." If the town did not clean up, the War Department would remove the troops.[68]

Women's clubs and church organizations took a particular interest in preventing the city's reputation from collapsing.[69] Philanthropist and clubwoman M. Eleanor Brackenridge stated, "San Antonio's good name has been called into question . . . and unless we do something, the stigma will be on our city. You men have begun the crusade and the women want to assist."[70] The crusade to clean up San Antonio took on a distinct gendered language, with women demanding increased activism in the public sphere as moral arbiters and as patriotic citizens. As one of the founders of the Woman's Club of San Antonio (WCSA), Brackenridge was a staunch supporter of women's rights, the war effort, and women's public role in moral protection. The club membership numbered more than five hundred in the 1910s, including "most ladies of social consequence." These were the women local politicians considered the appropriate voice of reform in the era.[71]

Members of the WCSA took it upon themselves to contribute to the war effort in whatever form they could, especially through the vice crusade. The clubwomen of San Antonio claimed as their own territory moral policing as a program of "municipal housekeeping," the idea that women's skills keeping a tidy and healthy house could be expanded to keeping cities clean. The *San Antonio Express* advocated this viewpoint, arguing that women's public role in the antivice campaign was an extension of their progressive role as defenders of public morality and a suitable way to contribute to the war effort. "The women of San Antonio have spoken on the vice situation. . . . By virtue of their sacrificial gifts they have the right to speak and to demand of their Government, National, State, and municipal, that the bodies and souls of their boys shall be protected." This editorial justified women's political activism based on the concept of patriotic motherhood.[72] Women's organizations and the churches took an active and vocal role in connecting moral policing with patriotism and the antivice campaign.

The women's cleanup campaign united local and national efforts. The War Department sent women social workers into the town in November 1917 with the goal of "guarding the morals of the young women of the community." They aimed to protect the health of the soldiers as well as protect the girls "against their own weakness more than anything else." It was the duty of mothers to provide moral stewardship for the young women seeking employment in town; girls lacking suitable mothers had to turn to alternate sources of moral guidance, be they clubwomen, social workers, or the YWCA. They wished to prevent these girls from drifting into prostitution. The article subtitle claimed that the women would "prevent possible evils in [a] social way," implying they could fight the "social evil," prostitution.[73]

The clubwomen claimed the moral high ground, contrasting feminine reform to San Antonio's male politicians who faced corruption charges over the vice crusade.[74] One local clergy member claimed that the Great War had brought a moral rebirth to a tired nation. "Bishop Capes said that instead of believing, as he was told recently, that this war would put civilization back 200 years, he believed it would put it forward 200 years." Changes made on the home front as a result of the war would advance the causes of social purity, prohibition, and the reformation of wayward girls.[75]

In an effort to further protective and purity aims, the women's clubs requested the appointment of policewomen. In 1900, the WCSA had successfully pushed for the appointment of the first police matron in town to monitor female prisoners at the city jail.[76] The WCSA believed increasing women's role in antivice work would lead to less corruption within the police force and would provide girls protection from sexual exploitation on the street. This Progressive crusade assumed women would bring an uncorrupted, nonpartisan moral purpose to the job.[77] Brackenridge and her colleagues lobbied the mayor, the city council, and the local press to support the appointment of policewomen to prevent immorality and vice. Their work came to naught, as the municipal government remained reluctant to employ women, especially at night, to walk the streets.[78]

With the advent of the war, the influx of soldiers and strangers, and the crackdown on vice, the movement for policewomen once again gathered momentum. Several women's groups joined together to organize a mass meeting for women on November 30, 1917, at which they voted to petition the city to appoint twelve policewomen. In the resolution the women stated, "We cannot be patient with the laxity or negligence of police administration in this regard. . . . We realize that not alone upon city officials but upon individual citizens—parents and homemakers, teachers of our schools, churches and social organizations, rests equal responsibility in this great concern."[79] Equating male political and police power with corruption, the clubwomen of San Antonio used stereotypes of women's incorruptibility to forward their own political activism, prevent the exploitation of the vulnerable, and secure job opportunities for a few.

Days later, the women's demand received a rather hesitant endorsement from the city executive branch. On December 4, 1917, Mayor Bell agreed to answer the demand of the Woman's City Committee and declared he would appoint female police officers. It was not until December 28, and after much hemming and hawing, that the appointments materialized. Afterward, Mayor Bell backed away from his previous endorsement and questioned the safety of unchaperoned women on the streets at night. The clubwomen responded that other cities had implemented the program successfully. In 1908 the first woman had been appointed with arrest power, in Portland, Oregon. Spurred by the wartime situation, New York City appointed female officers as well.[80]

An editorial in the *San Antonio Express* challenged the mayor's reservations but still downplayed the radical potential of appointing policewomen: "There is a definite place for some women police in our city. It's not a question of woman suffrage, nor of militant feminism. Outside of all politics and all parties, there is a moral and civic need for these women officers." Their role, the editorial claimed, would be preventative and would rely on women's natural role as savers of those on the edge of criminality.[81]

On December 28, the city commissioners appointed six women as "city policemen," for a trial term of sixty days. The WCSA, which provided recommendations to the city on whom to hire, touted the policewomen's moral character and dedication to the antivice campaign. The *San Antonio Express* noted that several spoke Spanish fluently, indicating the city's concern with the Mexican American population in the city.[82]

The municipal government argued that the policewomen should possess full police powers but expected from the outset that their duties would revolve around preventive work in the antivice crusade. The original six appointees were granted the power to arrest individuals, but both the municipal government and the media coverage stressed their responsibility and moral aptitude for preventing vice. The policewomen patrolled amusement parks, movie theaters, hotel lobbies, and the streets looking for unescorted girls out at night or couples "spooning" or "flirting."[83] The policewomen reportedly criticized the "incorrect dancing positions" of several couples at a local dance hall, noted overly dark movie theater balconies, and trailed but did not confront a soldier consorting with a "suspicious" woman.[84] An interview with Mrs. R. C. Hugman, the first appointee, added that "she doesn't think physical force is necessary for the kind of work she is to do," implying a divide between the more dangerous roles of male officers and the preventive, subordinate roles of female officers.[85]

The Woman's City Committee continued to agitate for an increased role in law enforcement for women. They asked to add fifteen volunteer policewomen to assist the city-appointed ones. They also desired to improve the public's respect for women officers: in response to the ridicule the policewomen received from the public, "a plea for your patience with the policewomen was made by Mrs. [Jane] Rippin. She said too much must not be expected at first, and that they must not be laughed at when they made mistakes." Rippin's comments suggest that, despite the support of the press and women's clubs, many still treated the policewomen as something of a joke.[86]

Even this tepid support for policewomen's preventive work did not last. On February 1, 1918, the city commissioners dismissed the policewomen well before their sixty-day trial period ended. Commissioner Lowther summed up the stance of the city government on the matter: "We have employed these women police since the sixth of the month, and they have been successful in making two arrests, two arrests of drunkards. I cannot see where they have been of any value to the city."[87] Mayor Bell said that he planned to continue employing a night matron for the city, but he replaced the policewomen with six male officers.

This sparked another controversy that stretched well beyond law enforcement into the politics of equality and social purity. Mrs. Rena M. Green of the Woman's City Committee wrote a letter to the editor of the San Antonio Express, declaring, "We are not citizens." She continued, "This morning we learn that all of the policewomen are dismissed. This action makes us realize, as we have often done before, that we cannot call ourselves citizens of San Antonio, that even at this time of stress when conditions look very critical as to the honor and good faith of our city, our services are not wanted." She continued, linking citizenship to suffrage: "it is a perfectly fine lesson to us, showing us the greater need of our organization, and a wonderful demonstration of the power of the ballot and of our helplessness without it."[88] Green made explicit the link between women's involvement in the war effort and their expected citizenship rights. If women were willing to contribute to the war effort through their work on the vice crusade, they should be entitled to a fair share of the respect and privileges any man serving in the Army would expect.

The Women's City Committee held a mass meeting to pass a resolution protesting the firing of the policewomen and calling for the appointment of a female expert to train and support policewomen.[89] They claimed that the policewomen, despite few arrests, actually had served the purpose they were appointed to perform: preventing vice. They noted several instances where young girls caught in compromising situations were reprimanded or sent home to their parents. The Women's City Committee argued that the municipal government had set the policewomen up to fail by giving them less authority than male officers and then dismissing them for not attaining the same results.

This was a common situation in newly emerging fields of women's employment. As was also the case with health inspection, law enforcement jobs for women were set up chiefly to deflect fear of sexual impropriety, and the female employees often met with resentment from male colleagues and a lack of support from their employers.[90] These jobs did not necessarily smooth the path to power for women. The example of the San Antonio policewomen demonstrates both the moral motivation behind the appointments and the male resistance to female political and legal authority.

If the policewomen were not making many arrests, the same was not true of their male counterparts. By mid-1918, the arrests for vice charges increased considerably under political pressure from the War Department. Arrests related to prostitution in Bexar County more than tripled between November and December of 1917 and then increased exponentially throughout early 1918.[91] Furthermore, coverage of vice arrests increased in both the local English-language and Spanish-language newspapers. Reporters stressed the lurid details of arrests and highlighted the race of the people involved, the presence of soldiers, or connections to liquor or gambling. The actual act of prostitution seemed less important to the media and to the police than the disorderliness of the people involved. One news report on vice arrests carried the subheading "Two Negresses Reported Troublesome."[92] The newspaper coverage raises questions about how law enforcement officials and the media defined "troublesome" and how this related to the racial and gender identity of the subjects.

An unofficial tally taken by the *San Antonio Express* in May reported that the vice squad arrested 425 persons during the preceding month. Of those arrests, 231 were men and 194 women. Of the men, 125 were white, 61 black, 43 Mexican, and 2 Chinese. The arrested women included 92 (presumably white) "Americans," 47 "Negresses," and 55 Mexicans. A majority of the women arrested were racial minorities. Besides the standard violations of city ordinances, gambling, and alcohol regulations, 22 of the women were "charged with being undesirables."[93]

The Spanish-language press covered the vice raids in much the same way as the *San Antonio Express*, including the race and gender of perpetrators in their stories. *La Prensa*, a San Antonio daily, maintained a column "from the office of the police," which covered the vice crackdown as well. In November 1917 it reported, "women detained for lustfulness."[94] Later in the month, it recorded the arrest of thirty-one black men and four black women during a raid "in the colored neighborhood."[95] The Spanish-language press periodically identified black perpetrators by their race, but it did not identify "Mexicans" as often as the white press did. Unlike the white press, the Spanish-language press was apparently hesitant to connect the Mexican American population with crimes like prostitution. The lack of racial identification in the press also could indicate that many Mexican Americans identified themselves as white, especially in a triracial community like San Antonio. Whites may not have accepted Mexican Americans as equals, but they recognized a racial hierarchical distinction between African Americans and Mexican Americans. Whites nonetheless assigned Mexican American women many of the same racial stereotypes they applied to African American women: hot-blooded, sexually precocious, and promiscuous.[96] Mexican Americans occupied a position that challenged the traditional southern racial hierarchy of white over black. Historian Neil Foley notes that Mexican Americans could not fully adopt a white identity, but they were "white enough to escape the worst features of the Jim Crow South."[97]

Mexican Americans' place in segregated Texas depended on numerous factors including class, English language ability, skin color, and perceived Spanish heritage. From this tenuous position, middle-class Mexican American institutions such as *La Prensa* may have tried to deflect attention from Mexican American criminal reports in hopes of aligning themselves with the white power structure by highlighting black misdeeds.

For all racial groups, the terminology of vice charges had changed dramatically by the middle of 1918. Prostitution-related charges in late 1917 focused on actions, such as "soliciting" or "keeping a bawdy house." By mid-1918 they shifted into terminology that focused more on identity. The docket books contained charges such as "being a common prostitute" and "being immoral," and the newspapers frequently listed the crimes of these women as being of a particular race or being "undesirable." Official charges, as noted in newspaper reports and in docket books, became less likely by 1918 to stress action and more likely to give a charge of identity, like "being of questionable character" or "being a common prostitute."[98] *La Prensa* reported in November of the arrest of "women of doubtful conduct," while two months later the terminology tended to reflect character rather than behavior: police detained "lustful women" or "ill women."[99] Increasingly, the media reported women arrested by describing who they were, not what they did. This implied that the women themselves, not their behaviors, were considered threatening.

Women could run afoul of the law based both on who they were and with whom they associated. Trial records indicate that consorting with soldiers had two consequences: it implied sexual promiscuity, and it increased the severity of that promiscuity by directly endangering the war effort. Depositions from the trial of Mrs. Annie Lacey, who was convicted of keeping a house of prostitution in late 1917, frequently mentioned the comings and goings of soldiers near her property. Witnesses for the prosecution noted the presence of "one soldier and woman who claimed to be married, and [an]other soldier and woman who claimed to be brother and sister" as suspicious behavior.[100] A promiscuous woman was "a worse menace" to the soldiers than a German.[101] The perception of women's sexuality had altered from sexual victims to threatening sexual aggressors.

By March, the rules had tightened further. The city passed new ordinances restricting drunkenness and loitering within the "white zone" around military camps. "Between noon Sunday and noon Monday five civilians were arrested for being drunk and nine women arrested for being immoral," wrote one reporter.[102] That same day, sixty-four "Negro women" were arrested for vagrancy in the company of seventy-five Negro soldiers.[103] The article reported that the women were all taken into custody and charged but none of the men were.[104]

In San Antonio, as in cities across the nation, arrested women faced the threat of long-term detention. The Live Oak Farm served as a detention center and venereal disease hospital for incarcerated women in the region. Created by a $15,000 appropriation from President Wilson's discretionary fund, the city purchased property and buildings in 1918 for the housing of female delinquents. The facility held up to one hundred women at a time, segregated by race and ethnicity into white, black, and Mexican dormitories. Compared to the Dorcas Home, the detention home for black girls in Houston, Live Oak Farm had an ample budget and good facilities, but it maintained many features of the more prison-like institutions. Inmates participated in two hours of housework and two hours of sewing a day and spent the rest of their time out of doors doing chores or taking supervised recreation. One report observed, "Good behavior was rewarded with special privileges. A high wire stockade surrounded the premises."[105] The institution had the support of many of the most influential Progressive organizations in town: the Woman's City Committee, the San Antonio Mission Home and Training Schools, the local juvenile court, and several local charities. Live Oak Farm represented the avant-garde in Progressive rehabilitation of sexual delinquents, combining medical treatment, education, vocational training, and strict discipline to achieve its goals.

Complementing the more punitive measures, educational campaigns also demonstrated the Progressive agenda in San Antonio. The YWCA took out an advertisement in the *Express* aimed at raising money for girls' educational work, specifically to develop sex education and social morality lecture programs aimed at women and girls heading to Europe for war work. "The need of this is great—as conditions in war-stricken Europe are appalling, and American girls must be protected."[106] Presumably respectable white American women needed protection from foreign sources of contagion as well as domestic threats.

The San Antonio Woman's Club launched Travelers' Aid societies to assist and educate young girls coming to the city without parental supervision. They also expanded their previous educational lectures. In December, they brought in a woman physician to lecture on eugenics, touching on the basics of reproduction and the significance of venereal diseases. In February, they held a roundtable discussion of the effects of war on women.[107] Educational programs such as these for YWCA volunteers and members of the WCSA demonstrate that protection work among white middle-class women was much different from the coercive efforts against more marginal women.

Gender played a central role in the ways San Antonio, and the nation, fought vice and provided sex education. The San Antonio middle-class clubwomen saw the vice crackdown as a way to exert moral and political authority, stop male sexual exploitation of women, give advice to the needy, and claim a more powerful role for themselves in war work and governance. Yet women's access to power through Progressive moral reform was severely limited. Their modest successes, such as the appointment of female police officers in San Antonio, met with scorn and were quickly rolled back by entrenched male politicians.

The national crackdown led to violations of the civil rights of more than fifteen thousand mostly working-class and minority girls and women, who were incarcerated without trial (and usually without charges) during and after the war.[108] The Progressive efforts to protect girls, supply medical treatment, and provide sex education and vocational opportunities to them were overshadowed by the more punitive elements of social control, which often hinged on the girls' racial identity. White girls arrested for sexual delinquency might expect rehabilitation and lessons in social hygiene, while nonwhite girls were shunted into inferior, prison-like facilities.

The attack on prostitution during World War I reconfirmed divisions between women, rather than bridging race and class divisions to form a common identity around gender. Some women chose to sacrifice more marginalized women in order to secure their own agenda or their own advancement within the male political structure.[109] Case studies in western cities like Los Angeles noted a broad mix of races confined to detention homes but found that detention disproportionately affected the working class. In Portland, Oregon, the class aspects were even more obvious: a woman could be released from the Cedars Detention Home by posting a thousand dollars bail.[110] The wealthy took care of their own. Class and respectability could easily trump gender when seeking common ground.

Foremost, the policing of sexuality deliberately centered the rhetoric of sexuality on women. Women presented a threat to the war effort through their unbridled sexuality. They did not have to be prostitutes or infected with venereal disease in order to pose a threat; their gender caused suspicion. Government-produced sex education pamphlets taught women the proper way to attain sexual respectability, using white characters and highlighting white middle-class or aspirational morality. Stereotypes that labeled women outside of the white middle class as sexually uncontrollable influenced the wartime policies regarding their education, treatment, and detention. These stereotypes worked to distance whites from other races and justify racist and segregationist policies. Racial stereotypes served as a symbolic attempt to demonstrate whites' sexual propriety. Sexual propriety represented status and citizenship; the lack of it entitled the state to intervene.[111]

Policewomen were caught in the middle of expected gender roles and the changing nature of women's political activism. They had yet to get the vote and or an equal voice in policy decisions. Many women hesitated to shed their gendered propriety or passionlessness in order to challenge male prerogative. By defining the problem as one of policing soldiers, authorities denied women power that went beyond moral or spiritual guidance. Policing young women allowed for more activism on the part of female reformers, but the focus on women also led to more violations of women's civil rights. The women who participated in the incarceration of other women may have thought they were contributing to the protection of girls and the war effort, but female reformers most often lacked access to policy-shaping positions. Without direct political power, women like Maude Miner, former head of the Committee for the Protection of Women and Girls, had little ability to change policies they recognized as unfriendly to women.

By November 1918, when the war ended in Europe, the divide between women's rights and men's prerogative in the matter of sexuality was in stark contrast to the vibrant expansion of women's political powers. The Nineteenth Amendment, ratified in 1920, gave white women the vote but did not even the playing field. Voting restrictions and other privileges based on race still existed, and the educational gaps between rich and poor; white, brown, and black; and male and female persisted. The war strengthened the movement for sex education, but it did not destroy stereotypes about sexuality and identity. Race and class, historically contentious subjects in medical and social discourses about sexuality, did not fade into the background when sex education expanded. Instead, sex education and sexual policing reinforced the standard of white middle-class expectation, despite myriad challenges from the postwar culture.

Chapter Seven

Sex Education in the 1920s

Secretary of the Navy and evangelical Christian Josephus Daniels had spent the war years fearful of providing soldiers sex education and prophylactics. So much so that the Navy practically went behind his back, allowing Assistant Secretary Franklin D. Roosevelt to sign the order to supply condoms while Daniels was away from his office. With the military moving forward to support broad sex hygiene programs, would the civilian world be far behind? Sex education in the wake of World War I proved to be an odd mix of continued wartime necessity and a domesticated "normalcy." While discussing sex became more acceptable in the media and the school curriculum, conservatives still feared female sexual agency and the perceived threat of nonwhite sexuality.

Immediately after the end of World War I, restricting sexuality presented a conundrum for military and civilian officials. In late 1918, the military recognized that sexual dangers for soldiers worsened immediately after combat ended. VD rates rose again among soldiers stationed abroad, possibly as a side effect of soldiers' increased idle time.[1] A pamphlet developed for civilians shortly after the Armistice noted:

> The War is Over! The last gun has been fired, the last bomb dropped, the last torpedo shot. But there is one enemy which has done more damage than the Germans ever thought of. This enemy is called the Venereal Diseases [*sic*]. The Government has been fighting them openly and energetically and much has already been done, but the battle is not yet over. It is a battle of peace times just as much as of war times.[2]

How would that battle be fought?

Demobilization

Military experts and policy makers suggested prophylaxis should expand into civilian life, to sustain the gains made under the American Plan. Colonel George Walker of the Medical Corps proposed that civilian society follow in the military's footsteps: "In all large cities, public stations should be run by the State Health Department. . . . They should not be called by any other name except their right name, 'Prophylactic Stations,' and distinctly they should not be a part of a hospital."[3] He displayed faith in the Progressive strategy of cure through education: "The opposition comes chiefly from those who are either ignorant of what the plan of procedure is, or who are guided by personal prejudice. When it is thoroughly explained, this attitude, wherever it may exist, generally vanishes."[4] Major Wilbur A. Sawyer of the Medical Corps concurred: "the war against Germany is over, but the war against venereal disease is only started." He highlighted the effectiveness of the military campaign to both prevent and treat infection through motion pictures like *Fit to Fight*, lectures, and law enforcement, and he urged the nation to continue to support such work. Furthermore, Sawyer praised the military's tough restrictions during demobilization, which refused any infected soldier release orders until a doctor declared him uninfected. "The army is being sent home clean. Will their communities make it easy or difficult for them to remain so?"[5] Raymond Fosdick's "Fit for Fighting—and After" discussed the importance of maintaining the morality and habits established in the Army once the soldiers returned home.[6] Even the previously reticent secretary of the Navy, Josephus Daniels, endorsed a continued campaign against venereal diseases: "One of the compensations for the tragedy of war is the fact that an enlightened public opinion is behind the organized campaign to protect the youth against venereal disease. The campaign begun in war to insure the military fitness of men for fighting is quite as necessary to save men for civil efficiency."[7] Military and civilian officials recognized the benefits of the wartime social hygiene programs and wished to continue them. They used the language of eugenics—efficiency and racial strength—to advocate the improvement of the nation. But not all races were the same in this view.

Racial stereotypes led to harsh restrictions on African American soldiers during demobilization. More than four hundred thousand black troops served in World War I, and many expected their service to translate into a greater claim to citizenship upon their return to civilian life.[8] Black ambition for equality raised fears among many whites expecting to maintain strict segregation. Whites feared that black soldiers, especially those who had served with their less-discriminating French allies, would expect equal treatment politically, economically, and socially. No fear loomed larger than the fear that black men in France had gained sexual access to French women and brought back a desire for interracial liaisons.

The military command quickly acted to prevent interracial relationships in Europe. Captain Byrne, a white officer of the 804th Pioneer Infantry, an African American unit, released the following order on March 20, 1919: "Enlisted men of this organization will not talk to or be in company of any white women, regardless of whether the women solicit their company or not."[9] Two black YMCA workers, Addie Hunton and Kathryn Johnson, deplored the racial motivations behind such orders. They believed that the military designed the order to limit the behavior of the black soldiers as well as to convince the nearby civilians that blacks were "villains." Hunton and Johnson proudly reported, however, that the French citizens formed their own, usually positive, opinions about the black soldiers: "They gradually discovered that the colored American was not the wild, vicious character that he had been represented to be, but that he was kindhearted, genteel, and polite."[10] The YMCA directors published a letter they received from the mayor of Challes-les-Eaux, Savoie, after the Armistice. The mayor used language that infantilized the black soldiers but also praised them: "These black soldiers . . . are wonderful children, with generous hearts, a spirit of good comradeship, possessing also a French trait—that of loving and making themselves beloved."[11] Hunton and Johnson argued that French civilians disapproved of the white US military command's punitive treatment of black soldiers. Many French women refused to follow the American military instructions, claiming "they were the mistresses of their own homes and morals, and knew with whom they wished to associate, and did not desire American officers to interfere with their social affairs."[12] The order demonstrated the US military's fear of interracial sexual liaisons and of French women's reputed sexual freedom. French women could not be trusted, as their white American counterparts could, to refuse the attentions of black soldiers.[13]

Concern over women's sexual behavior continued on the home front as well. Local governments maintained detention homes after the Armistice, although not necessarily the educational programs they hosted. Social worker Martha P. Falconer wrote in 1918 that she hoped a permanent program would emerge out of the wartime necessity: "The problem of delinquency among women and girls, which we face today as menacing our military strength, is a problem which our awakening social conscience must face, in a lesser degree, in times of peace."[14] Many of the institutions funded by the federal government operated into the 1920s. Some sought to maintain operations through philanthropic donations after federal money dried up. The arrests decreased after the Armistice, but authorities did not completely stop arresting women, nor did they release their inmates upon demobilization.[15]

Detention homes continued operations as long as they could find funding. Live Oak Farm in San Antonio continued to receive funding from the city in 1919, and ASHA's publication, the *Journal of Social Hygiene*, used it as an example of how municipalities should maintain these facilities.[16] But in August 1920, the city shut it down and transferred the inmates to the city jail. In jail, any educational programs that Live Oak maintained fell by the wayside. This pattern repeated across the nation. The Cedars detention center in Portland, Oregon, was closed in 1923 because of lack of funding. Portland clubwomen did not oppose detention itself but wanted more equality between the genders. They urged the city to open a similar institution for men and to appoint more female doctors and board members to the Cedars administration.[17] Los Feliz, a detention facility for women in Los Angeles, finally closed in 1924. But until then the "Purity Squad," an undercover police unit, continued to arrest and detain women suspected of infection.[18] Eventually, the money simply ran out to continue detention.[19]

Without federal funding, who would fill the budgetary gap to pay for social hygiene programs? Armistice did not immediately end the military's concern over sex, nor did it resolve the national debate over social hygiene. ASHA hoped that the focus on education rather than detention would ensure the organization's future in the uncertain days following the Armistice. The Chamberlain-Kahn Act, which allotted $2 million to promote VD eradication and sex education programs, passed in 1918, but funding declined rapidly by 1922.[20] ASHA's annual budget dropped from $335,000 in 1919 to $200,000 in 1923.[21]

But a renewed emphasis on education drew the attention of education- and public health–minded philanthropists. Under the direction of Katherine Bement Davis, the Rockefeller Foundation's Bureau of Social Hygiene provided financial support to ASHA to continue its work. Rockefeller offered to match contributions, providing two dollars for every one ASHA raised, up to $100,000. The Bureau of Social Hygiene wanted to parlay "emergency" measures into a permanent endeavor. A letter from the early 1920s sent to contributors read, "As the ultimate object of the Association is the protection of the family through wise sex education, the repression of prostitution, and the reduction of the venereal diseases, emphasis is being placed this year on education."[22] Davis supported continued scientific research into human sexuality, as well as more robust education. If the renewed emphasis was education, what should be taught and how?

The New Normalcy

Many historians have described the 1920s in the inventive words of President Warren Harding: a "return to normalcy."[23] After the social, political, and demographic upheaval of World War I, many Americans were all too willing to forget the thorny issues brought up by Progressive reform and concentrate instead on business as usual. The reactionary policies of the federal government, which sought to silence dissent during and after the war through legal and sometimes extralegal means, facilitated this response.[24] The positive presentation of "normalcy" and the growing prosperity of the 1920s allowed many people to practice middle-class consumer patterns that had been out of reach.

Normalcy was not just a political or economic movement. To many Americans, normalcy represented a comforting cultural standard. But was the culture the same as before the war? After World War I, Americans continued to accept increasingly frank sexual discourse and behaviors, institutionalizing the sexual "revolution" of the war years. Social scientists, researchers, and educators turned their attention from vice and VD to establishing a definition of what constituted—and how to attain—a "normal" sex life. Many white reformers shifted their aims from antiprostitution efforts to assisting unwed mothers, often working under the mistaken assumption that prostitution had disappeared. Yet, in reality, prostitution often was pushed out of the "white zones" into racially segregated neighborhoods, both North and South.[25] Whites saw interracial sex as a sign of societal degeneracy and a threat to racial strength and purity.[26] The ominous fear of interracial sex helped bolster segregation in the southern states, while white consumers could enjoy the erotic fantasy constructed around "savage" black sexuality in the jazz scene of Harlem and other northern urban centers.[27] The United States was a nation divided by race, by class, by gender, by region, and by generation.

Despite its best efforts, segregating sexuality never fully worked. The public battle over "khaki fever" and sexual delinquency indicated that the nineteenth-century idealization of female "passionlessness" had lost its force. Of course, that did not stop many experts from reverting to Victorian beliefs. The US Public Health Service's exhibit, *Keeping Fit*, showcased prewar assumptions by presenting women as victims of men's sexual degeneracy. One poster, for instance, showcased a rosy-cheeked young woman with the caption, "This girl may become an invalid for life if she marries a man who has gonorrhea not entirely cured." Nowhere does the exhibit, aimed at men, address female sexual agency. Instead, the assumption was that women (at least, good women) entered marriage with "honor and purity" and it was men's duty to be worthy of that purity.[28] *Keeping Fit* chose reticence to shore up its middle-class ideal self-control and purity.[29]

The Public Health Service poster series aimed at girls, *Youth and Life*, combined scientific elements of sex education with odd messages about women's sexuality. "The secretion of the ovaries makes the girl grow into a woman," reads one placard alongside a picture of a girl picking an apple. The next poster reads, "Sex endows the girl with beauty of body, vivacity, and charm of manner. It is the sex or creative impulse which inspires her warmth of affection, her intensity of purpose, her desire to devote herself to the welfare of humanity." Puberty thus makes a woman ready to be motherly toward her children and the world, but not to have sexual desires. She may not be passionless, but her passions were far from sexual.[30] Maintaining the practice of segregation of health education, the US Public Health Service adapted the *Keeping Fit* series in 1920 for African American boys and considered developing one for African American girls as well.[31] The Public Health Service sold or loaned out lantern slides and pamphlets based on the posters throughout the 1920s. Their slides, though, rarely went beyond the old model of female protection and male honor, except that it implied that African Americans required separate (if similar) lessons. Of course, the *Keeping Fit* version for African Americans merely swapped out images of whites for images of blacks.[32]

Despite the government's efforts, sex education material that focused on women's passionlessness failed to sway audiences as it had a decade before.[33] In fact, some sex hygiene books of the 1920s ridiculed the previous generation's books, noting their outdated sexual standards and calls to religious authority. The popular Sex and Self series by Sylvanus Stall, published continuously since 1897, seemed too steeped in conservative religiosity. William J. Fielding, author of sex education titles for the affordable Little Blue Notebook series in the 1920s, attempted to market his work against Stall's by accusing Stall of encouraging shame about sexuality. Fielding titled his series Rational Sex, using modern parlance, and declared sex "the very foundation of life, health and happiness," not something to be feared.[34]

Americans in the 1920s recognized that many women of all races and classes were having and enjoying sex.[35] Containing and controlling sexuality, rather than denying it, formed the backbone of the postwar curriculum. Education turned from pathologizing sex to establishing proper marital adjustment. Colleges across the nation implemented marital life courses, designed to prepare young men and women for healthful heterosexual relationships.[36] Led by formal institutions that catered to the middle class, the 1920s sex education curriculum, whether it came from ASHA, the schools, or the medical profession, focused on asserting white middle-class norms. Educators pounced on the new psychology of the 1920s to argue why premarital sex would damage proper sexual adjustment after marriage. The end result: lessons that accepted the importance of sexual fulfillment but stressed waiting until marriage.[37]

The US Public Health Service attempted to take an active role in guiding sex education in the 1920s. It produced two reports, in 1922 and 1927, giving modern readers a glimpse into the spread of sex education in the 1920s. While the surveys returned did not represent a random sample, they reported that 40–45 percent of high school seniors had some exposure to sex education.[38] Mostly, high schools that offered sex education in their curriculum did so through biology classes, adding human reproduction, heredity, and eugenics into the curriculum. But by 1927, more social studies classes were tackling the social aspects of sex education, including monogamy, attraction, and relationships. Large urban schools were more likely to (and more capable of) offering sex education. The South lagged behind both the North and the West, similar to the regional differences experienced in the early days of ASHA and the social hygiene movement. Without local community interest, sex education curricula could easily disappear.[39] Outside of biology and social studies classes, the newly popular physical education courses offered a new home for sex education.

Physical education classes gained in popularity after the war because of the military concern over health and wellness. The classes were usually segregated by sex (and often by race, since many schools were segregated) in high schools and colleges. Assumptions about the fundamental differences between males and females, especially women's menstrual cycles, provided all the justification needed to separate males and females in gym class. Female physical education instructors served as experts who not only guided girls through socially appropriate exercises but also provided an ear to hear problems and a voice to teach students about their health and bodies.[40]

Outside of schools, health and wellness programs also flourished. The Girl Scouts of America instituted the Health Winner Badge in the 1920s, which required a girl to learn the physiology of menstruation and have a private talk with her troop leader. One of the main motivations behind this was to shield the girl from overexerting herself during her period.[41] While the Girl Scouts maintained that ideally the girl would turn to her mother or physician to learn about her body, the organization worried that too many girls lacked someone knowledgeable and willing to discuss such topics. The Girl Scouts' policies depict a generational change; what was appropriate discussion for the younger generation may not have been to the prewar generation.

Sex education publishing expanded during the 1920s, as more books were published to both get information across to audiences and to make a profit. The expanding market demonstrated increased interest the topic. Comparing William J. Fielding's sex education books to those of Sylvanus Stall's generation demonstrates a changing frankness.[42] Margaret Sanger continued publishing into the 1920s, expanding on her prewar work on birth control and women's and workers' rights. Added to her old arguments, Sanger also supported family limitation to counter "the reactionaries demanding a higher and still higher birth rate" to support "militaristic tendencies." Reducing family size would not only help women economically and politically but would stave off future wars.[43] Sanger continued providing a radical voice for sex education and women's rights, although her socialistic leanings disappeared in her later writings.[44]

Besides the nonfiction publishing world, fiction provided another path to sexual knowledge, as writers like F. Scott Fitzgerald celebrated—and helped create—the sexually adventurous flapper who symbolized the 1920s. Perhaps one of the biggest changes in the 1920s was the publication of Radclyffe Hall's *The Well of Loneliness* in 1928. Scholar Lillian Faderman describes the publication of Hall's novel as the first forthright lesbian literature widely available in the United States. The novel portrays lesbianism (called sexual inversion) as natural and neutral in value. Hall used her novel to popularize the ideas of sexologists like Krafft-Ebing and Havelock Ellis, thus reaching a far wider audience than they had.[45] Despite efforts to have it banned both in Hall's native England and the United States, the book found a broad audience and became a topic of much conversation.

The lessons of sex education expanded from the military and character-building organizations to the public schools and the popular press. The prosperity and urban life of the 1920s allowed more young people to attend high school and even college.[46] For both working-class and middle-class youth, peer culture and popular culture took the place of the long-standing traditions of family and faith as their primary identity. Students gained their knowledge about sexuality as much from their interaction with their friends as they did from formal educational approaches. The media both contributed to and publicized this revolution.[47]

Sex in Popular Culture: Alternate Classrooms of the Roaring Twenties

Sexual knowledge has always been communicated outside of printed literature or official curricula, and in the 1920s, that became all the more apparent. The obscenity laws that remained so overarching during the Progressive Era fell out of fashion after the death of Anthony Comstock, whose name gave us the Comstock Laws. Movies, literature, and entertainments provided ample evidence of an awakening sexual culture tied inextricably to commercial entertainment.

Motion pictures formed the backbone of commercial entertainment in the postwar era. Following in the footsteps of lantern slide and stereopticon shows, educators used film to get their messages across to both the military and civilian populations. But the war changed the organized response to film censorship as well.

While there had been isolated protests against films that depicted white slavery, venereal diseases, and birth control prior to the war, it was the response to *Fit to Fight* and *The End of the Road*, the military-sponsored sex hygiene films, around which protestors coalesced. Members of the Catholic Church formed the National Catholic War Council in 1917 to challenge the CTCA and the American Plan. While both Catholics and Protestants were concerned with the themes of the war film, it was Catholic priest Father John J. Burke who spearheaded censorship efforts.[48]

While Catholics were certainly not unanimous in their disapproval of "smutty" films, the hierarchy of the Catholic Church encouraged organizing and threatened a boycott. The potential loss of twenty million Catholics, most located in urban centers where most of the nation's movie theaters were located, was too much for Hollywood to ignore. They had to listen, and the voices they listened to were often Catholic. Figures like Joseph Breen, Daniel Lord, and Martin Quigley shaped the debate throughout the 1920s on Hollywood censorship.[49]

According to the Motion Picture Producers and Distributors of America, "No picture shall be produced that will lower the moral standards of those who see it." The Hays Code argued that arts and entertainment, including film, provided "important influences in the life of a nation" and therefore filmmakers and distributers needed to be mindful of the moral messages of their films.[50] The producers of educational sex hygiene films argued that the films taught important lessons. Censors argued that they merely titillated audiences, and the Hays Code specifically banned sex hygiene films. This inclusion into the code likely resulted from the practice of filmmakers to reward chastity and punish sexuality in the end as a way to get around accepted standards of decency. For example, "white slavery" films of the 1910s and 1920s were often made more to titillate, but tacked on a moral and proper ending in order to avoid charges of indecency.

The National Catholic Welfare Conference (the peacetime continuation of the National Catholic War Council) battled two sex hygiene films in 1919, *Know Thy Husband* and *Open Your Eyes*. Both were VD message films, supposedly intent on teaching young people to recognize the medical and moral dangers of premarital sex and avoid marriage with dissipated men. *Know Thy Husband* actually suggests that syphilis could be cured quite easily, an overly optimistic scenario in the days before penicillin. National Catholic Welfare Conference film reviewer Charles McMahon, who reported directly to Father Burke, argued that the film's presentation of "knowledge of the possible consequences of evil did not dissuade anybody but apparently made people more determined to try it themselves." He concluded that the films were not aiming to educate or improve people but just to "exploit the topic in order to make money."[51]

Yet there was more to film censorship than simply reducing explicit sexuality. The Hays Code also forbade miscegenation, censoring any depiction of romantic relationships between the races. Hollywood miscegenation was a threat to white supremacy in the same way as contact between black soldiers and French women during World War I. Interracial sex threatened both the hard lines of white supremacy and the eugenic attitudes of racial purity. Throughout the early days of the movie industry, concern about what was on the screen also reflected concern over who was in the audience. Movie theaters were places where working-class, immigrant, and mixed-race audiences gathered together, in the dark, without chaperones. Centered in large, diverse cities, movie theaters represented the fears of the unbridled sexuality of the city as much in what was off the screen as on. Any real challenge to the racial hierarchy was just as threatening as the possibility of seduction on the silver screen.

In the midst of the Great Migration, urban centers like Harlem, in New York City, formed the locus of the new opportunity for seduction in the 1920s. During the Harlem Renaissance, whites sought out speakeasies and jazz clubs that allowed them to witness, or participate in, a "different" kind of sexuality without damaging their own respectability.[52] Both restriction and exotic fantasy deepened the alleged divide between white and nonwhite sexualities. The blues gave voice to female agency in sexuality, including the possibility of homosexual behavior, through the work of artists like Ma Rainey and Gladys "Fatso" Bentley, offering audiences another way of learning about alternate sexualities.[53]

More concrete than the vagaries of artistic performance, middle-class women's magazines like *Good Housekeeping* and *Redbook* began advertising feminine hygiene products. In 1921, the *Ladies Home Journal* ran an ad for Kotex menstrual pads invoking World War I as a motivation for improved feminine hygiene products. Next to an image of a military nurse, the text read, "Necessity being the mother of invention, our war nurses in France first discovered a new use for Cellucotton, which has led to Kotex."[54] Many of the Kotex ads included an address customers could write to should they have questions or want a sample of the product. By advertising in middle-class magazines, Kotex spoke indirectly to the class identity of their customer base; directly, the ad copy claimed, "Kotex is used by eight women in ten in the better walks of life."[55] In 1929, Kotex also celebrated women's newfound freedom from the limits of their monthly difficulties: "'Marvelous . . . the freedom with this new sanitary protection.' says an outdoor girl." Advertisements stressed the peace of mind schoolgirls, adventurous girls, and office girls all could gain through better knowledge (and better products). Kotex promised "health first" to customers who ordered their product, noting "four reasons why doctors recommend Kotex to all women" and offering a "valuable book on women's hygiene—Free."[56] Kotex ads claimed the approval not just of women's magazines but also women doctors and nurses.[57] A new consumer culture spread throughout the 1920s, inundating audiences with sexual information—and occasional explicit sex education—from the silver screen, the phonograph, and the newsstand.

By the dawn of the 1920s, the nation had started a new chapter in its development: the development of a new "normalcy," forever changed by the catalyst of war. World War I had strengthened both the public acceptance of sex education as a necessity and the federal government's involvement in health matters. The Eighteenth Amendment, enacting Prohibition, reflected a fear of perceived immoral (often immigrant) culture, but it also demonstrated the willingness of the federal government to attempt to legislate and enforce morality. Like the antivice campaigns of the 1910s, the antialcohol movement of the 1920s may have done little more than push vice into an underground (and attractive) economy.[58] Reformers had long tied prostitution and sexual permissiveness to drinking, so it is not surprising that Prohibition and anti vice were often linked. The dry Victorians and the wet flappers represented a generational divide over drinking and hemlines, but also over new attitudes toward sexual frankness.

It seemed clear that a greater sexual permissiveness tied in both the media and the younger generation. Unable to fully put the genie back in the bottle, reformers tried to domesticate sex education, urging premarital abstinence to ensure better sexual satisfaction in marital life. High schools and college experimented with sex hygiene courses geared toward healthy heterosexual marriage; physical education and health curricula celebrated keeping fit, catalyzed by the wartime emergency. The Victorian era was dead, but not without a few dying gasps. Whether it was movie producers walking a thin line between education and entertainment, anxiety about race mixing in classrooms or amusements, or civilian communities continuing to imprison suspected prostitutes, efforts to control sexual hierarchies through sex education were hard to shake.

Conclusion

In 1901, ASHA's founding voice, Prince Morrow, lamented the unnecessary hostility between purity reformers and the medical community. In the twenty-first century, that hostility still exists. A century after the founding of ASHA, the debate over sex education in the United States has not calmed. While in the 1920s, sex education found its way into many high schools and colleges, often in the form of preparing students for heterosexual marriage, resistance to it never disappeared. Sex education was domesticated throughout the mid-twentieth century, segregated by gender and often by race, stressing the value of heterosexual marriage. Then, once again, in the shadow of greater challenges to rigid social hierarchies, political forces pushed back against sex education.

Where Is the Revolution?

Many historians have pushed back the American sexual revolution from the 1920s or the 1960s to the 1910s.[1] Restructuring the timeframe is crucial to understanding the early sex education movement. Prince Morrow and ASHA employed quintessentially Progressive strategies to manage sexual knowledge. He and his allies did not radically challenge existing standards of sexual morality but assumed that men were sexually aggressive, white women passive, and nonwhites problematic subjects for proper education. But Morrow and ASHA held fast to the Progressive optimism that most people could be taught to control their sexual impulses if only more information were available.

Efforts to introduce ASHA's message to the world, especially through the public schools, proved problematic. Progressives demanded that some institution fill the gap, because they doubted parents' ability or willingness to teach the subject. A morality-based sex education curriculum, circulated by nondenominational Christian organizations such as the YMCA and the Boy Scouts, blended chivalry, sexual health, and manliness to form a white middle-class ideal. The character-building organizations that appropriated the social hygiene movement largely abandoned women, the poor, and racial minorities.

Outside of the white male ideal, the rhetoric surrounding sex education became far more cynical. The intense medical and social scrutiny of race at the turn of the century damaged social hygiene programs that crossed the color line. White southern physicians suggested that any educational efforts for African Americans would be hopeless, while African Americans dared to challenge stereotypes, creating their own programs to prevent disease and uplift the race.

The wartime draft supplied the first reliable VD rates, proving that VD was a national, not racial, problem. The government's Progressive ideology, represented by policy makers like Wilson, Baker, and Fosdick, sacrificed the code of silence for concerted action out of military necessity. A two-pronged strategy emerged to police dangerous sexual behavior. The War Department urged soldiers to maintain their chastity in the name of the war effort. The military and local police punished female civilians severely for "menacing" soldiers. Besides the divide between men and women, more subtle class and race distinctions further distanced the salvageable sinner from the enemy within. Anglo white girls received sex education and vocational training, while African American and Mexican American girls were held in prison-like conditions with little effort at education or rehabilitation.

The "return to normalcy" of the 1920s may have been the death knell for Progressivism, but the ultimate triumph of sex education after World War I was its normalization. However, the accepted hierarchies, which placed the white middle class on a pedestal and supported male sexual prerogative over female sexual expression, held fast after the Armistice.

Authorities and experts used sex education during the Progressive Era and World War I to divide rather than unite people. Medical "expertise" about the danger of venereal disease supported racial segregation and limited education in the South. In contrast, black physicians used scientific knowledge and sex education to challenge segregation and to establish their own expertise and respectability. Working-class and minority women during World War I found themselves on the defensive, and fifteen thousand were placed in detention centers for fear of the spread of venereal diseases to military men. But some feminist voices argued that frank sex education—equally distributed to men and women—was the only solution.

Not surprisingly, the militarized rigidity of sexual hierarchies did not die after World War I. Questionable sexual health assumptions popped up a generation later during the struggle to end segregation. After President Harry Truman's order to desegregate the military in 1948, Senator Richard Russell of Georgia argued that whites should not have to serve with blacks, since Russell claimed blacks had an "appallingly high" rate of venereal disease.[2] Politicians and military officials have made similar arguments about the dangers of opening up the military to women, who brought with them the danger of pregnancy and sexually transmitted diseases, and openly gay men, due to fear of HIV/AIDS.

In 2013, military debates over the failure to report or prosecute sexual assault against both men and women in the military led some conservatives to doubt whether that men and women could serve successfully together, because of teens' raging hormones, of course. Georgia Representative Saxby Chambliss, while decrying the culture of assault that seems to surround the military, argued, "The young folks that are coming into each of your services are anywhere from 17 to 22–23. Gee whiz—the hormone level created by nature sets in place the possibility for these types of things to occur."[3] This justified efforts to roll back women's gains in the military and to suggest that men and women could not serve successfully together. More traditional hierarchical relations between men and women, heterosexual and homosexual people, and whites and nonwhites have apparently not disappeared from military or civilian society. Scientific and cultural "norming" of whiteness, masculinity, and heterosexuality is invisible, yet ever present. And those norms reinforce the power of white heterosexual men.[4] On the issue of sexual assault, sex education curricula has often taught girls how best to avoid rape but not taught boys the importance of consent. We are still working with the faulty notion that women do not seek out sex (and if they do, they deserve victimization) while boys are animals who cannot resist their insatiable sex drives.

In the wake of the *Brown v. Board of Education of Topeka* case in 1954, conservative whites resisted school desegregation using rhetoric about the menace of (sexual) race mixing, that school segregation would undoubtedly lead to interracial sexual liaisons.[5] White supremacists capitalized on the trope that supposedly oversexed black boys would be in close proximity to white girls. The collapsing hierarchies of race worked not just on a black-white dichotomy, but among Latinos, Asians, and Native Americans as well. Pablo Mitchell's work on sex crimes in the American Southwest in the early twentieth century highlights the importance of strict sexual segregation as the only way to maintain clear lines of who is white and who is not. At a time when Mexican Americans were struggling to hold onto a "middle rung" between white and black America, the potential for miscegenation complicated what was already a slippery slope of racial identity.[6] The notion of sexual assault in mixed-race settings worked both ways, as Danielle McGuire's work reframes the civil rights movement through the lens of sexual assault and protection of black women.[7] The Chicano movement and American Indian movement both had to cope with sexualized stereotypes that were used as excuses to maintain rigid racial hierarchies, including white men's sexual access to marginalized women.

In addition to civil rights for racial minorities, the women's liberation movement of the 1960s thoroughly challenged basic assumptions related to sex education. Consciousness-raising groups created grassroots pressure for sex education while challenging both school curricula and the medical establishment. Perhaps the best example of this is the Boston Women's Health Book Collective, formed in 1969 out of a women's liberation group's discussion of women's health issues. This truly revolutionized sex education, reorienting expertise to the experience of ordinary women. The collective gathered essays on birth control, breastfeeding, menstruation, menopause, lesbianism, and much more, from medical, emotional, and experiential perspectives. They eventually turned their newsprint pamphlets into a commercially available book, *Our Bodies, Ourselves*, which has been updated, revised, and reprinted regularly for the past forty years.[8]

The backlash against the 1960s protest movements triggered a resurgence of political conservatism, which took sex education in American schools as one of its main foes. The New Right made sex education a foremost example of "liberal permissiveness." Conservatives placed anti-sex-education agitation within a larger context of culture wars and Cold War suburban politics. New Right activists categorized the public schools' sex education curriculum as a symbol of feminism, civil rights, communism, and the breakdown of Christian, middle-class values.[9] The right-wing reaction against sex education, complete with fabrications about and exaggerations of the curriculum, was a response more to the sexual revolution of the 1960s than it was to the retrenched, limited education students received in the classroom. Rather than arguing for a complete removal of sex education, late twentieth-century conservative activists instead proposed new curricula more in keeping with their values.[10]

Supporters and opponents of sex education continue to claim "scientific truth" to further their moral agendas. The late twentieth-century "abstinence-only" education speaks to recurring fears over cultural values, religion, and women's place in society. Abstinence-only curricula often present outdated gender stereotypes as scientific facts and present misleading or inaccurate data to encourage abstinence. These tactics are similar to those employed by educators in the 1910s, who often used pseudoscientific scare tactics to ensure compliance to traditional models of sexual reticence. William J. Robinson's 1916 textbook decried the way other authors, even those who claimed scientific authority, included "lurid exaggerations or downright falsehoods" to scare audiences into abstinence.[11] Many educators were then and are now willing to trade scientific accuracy for their desired outcomes.[12] For example, experts manipulated the rates of venereal disease infection, which had never been accurately measured before World War I, to favor their own political agendas; a low rate suggested that there was no need to change the status quo regarding education or behavior, while a high rate suggested the need for radical change. Purity reformers won the day in the 1990s, establishing tax funding for with the establishment of "abstinence-only" curricula for public schools, but with questionable results.[13]

The messages behind the science of sexuality have always contained a political angle. Indeed, access to sexual knowledge itself has been a feminist cause for a century, even if that was not the original aim of male doctors.[14] Clelia Duel Mosher and Margaret Sanger advocated women's increased knowledge as a vital part of women's emancipation from patriarchal control in the 1910s. Sex education served a far broader purpose than merely teaching people to stay healthy. It provided access to health information without the requirement of an intermediary, which allowed women and racial minorities to sidestep white male "experts," a crucial step in establishing their physical and political autonomy. But individual rights were not necessarily human rights. The intersection of feminism and racial equality has been tenuous, as many of the feminist thinkers of the early twentieth century, like the policewomen in San Antonio, scapegoated nonwhites in an attempt to shore up their own power.

The demands for scientifically accurate medical information about sex have repeatedly run into a brick wall of moralizing. While efforts to maintain social hierarchies of race are (usually) no longer blatant, political power assumed by the Religious Right and the accepted gender norms of the white evangelical movement, continue to shape policy, sometimes to the detriment of scientifically sound information. Issues related to gender and especially heterosexual norms are still contested in character-building organizations like the Boy Scouts. The front-and-center viewpoints of religious organizations continue to define through their political proxies who is and who is not salvageable.

The nineteenth-century notion that sexually transmitted diseases or unwanted pregnancies were God's punishment for sin lingers with us. Surgeon General C. Everett Koop's discussion of the AIDS crisis of the 1980s raised the ire of religious conservatives. Conservatives believed they could count on Koop, President Ronald Reagan's appointment to the surgeon general position, to hold firm to traditional, religious viewpoints. Koop, however, surprised both his supporters and his opponents by presenting explicit, accurate information on the transmission of AIDS and urging greater education (including a Public Health Service pamphlet sent out in the largest mass mailing in American history) to prevent its spread. His forthright advice and unwillingness to moralize about homosexuality—he repeatedly stated he had to separate the "Christian" from the "physician"—caused conservatives like William Buckley and Phyllis Schlafly to denounce him. The federal Public Health Service under Koop carefully used neutral and clinical terms to avoid moral judgments, while still expressing the dangers of promiscuity. Koop advocated both abstinence and condoms, giving a surprisingly nuanced approach to sex education.[15]

In the twenty-first century, it seems issues of sexuality are never far from the twenty-four hour news cycle. Antiabortion politicians got into hot water in an attempt to weed out pregnancies resulting from consensual sex from those resulting from rape, where there is a wide consensus that abortion should be an option. In 2012, Missouri Representative and Senate candidate Todd Akin was interviewed on the topic of banning abortion. When discussing the issue of an exception for rape victims, he stated, "First of all, from what I understand from doctors, that's really rare. If it's a legitimate rape, the female body has ways to try to shut that whole thing down." Akin's claim of scientific expertise via his purported consultation with a doctor was immediately attacked for being not just scientifically inaccurate but also harmful to women's bodily autonomy. Feminists argued that he was claiming either that rape could be

divided into categories of "legitimacy" (as he clarified later, "forcible" rape versus nonforcible) or he was suggesting that women lied about rape in order to
procure abortions. Akin's statements went viral across all media, contributing
to his loss in the senate race in the fall of 2012.[16] While scientifically accurate
information is available regarding pregnancy rates from rape, too often people
who either do not know or do not care what the science says are the ones shaping policy.

Despite the enduring pattern of morality versus scientific accuracy, there is
one modern revolution that has taken hold: the Internet. Adults, teens, and
children can access a riot of information on sexuality with only an Internet
connection. They can search the web for answers to their questions about their
bodies, their desires, and their behaviors. Like in the early twentieth century,
new media provides a degree of "gee whiz" that appeals to a wide swath of
people. On the Internet, users can access a variety of information about sex, as
well as graphic (or pornographic) images and videos. Access to sexual information may no longer be a problem for most Americans, but determining what is
accurate versus inaccurate information is perhaps harder than ever. One of the
main issues educators and health professionals face in the twenty-first century
is students or patients who view all information found online as equally reasonable and useful. Critical evaluation of material—the establishment of expertise—is still required.

Sex education in the early twentieth century had the potential to provide
people with the knowledge necessary to keep them healthy, safe, and satisfied.
Instead, it was often limited or denied for fear of awakening the danger of adolescent or nonmarital sexuality. To complicate matters even further, sometimes
it was provided in such limited and misleading ways that it was used to reinforce pernicious stereotypes about gender, race, or class categories. We want
to believe that so much has changed, that the hierarchies and stereotypes of
the past are gone. But has it? Are we still seeing education as a way of trying to
either empower people through knowledge or resisting the possibility of grant-
ing everyone the same education—the same knowledge/power that might
allow for a more equitable solution?

Sex, so intricately connected to American assumptions about gender, race,
and class, meant more than just what went on in the bedroom. Consider
two contrasting lessons from the Fourth International Congress on School
Hygiene, held in 1913. G. Stanley Hall, the eminent psychologist and founder
of the modern study of adolescence, wrote, "Every man should be just as manly
and every woman just as womanly as possible. It is vital to the race that sex distinction, which primitive and savage life often rather tends to obscure, should
be pushed to their uttermost. The highly civilized woman and man differ more
and more from each other in bodily dimensions, in life occupation, in mental,
moral, social traits."[17] At the same conference, Robert Willson argued, "Our
women and children are not free! We must regain that cherished title, and in

order to succeed we must redeem ourselves before our own conscience by first placing woman where she belongs, on a plane of social and moral and political equality with men."[18] Both men advocated sex education, but for different purposes. Hall wished to ensure the continued separation of the sexes, as befit a racially specific "advanced civilization." Willson wished to grant women greater equality through active participation in all aspects of life. Progressive educators hoped that the lessons of sex education would contribute to the fulfillment of a person's role in society. Debate over what that role should be, defined and delineated by race, class, and gender, inexorably shaped the curriculum.

The Progressive Era efforts at establishing sex education was a product of its time—reform oriented rather than revolutionary, tied to traditional assumptions of social control and expertise, and unwilling to beat back the hierarchies of race, class, and gender in American life. Radicals like Margaret Sanger and Robert Willson were stymied by the Comstock Laws, as well as their more moderate allies in ASHA and other reform organizations. Sex hygiene in the public schools—well, people simply were not ready for it. Even in the 1920s, the supposed flapper generation of easy virtue and emancipated women, sex education was domesticated into marriage training classes, reasserting both heteronormativity and conservative values.

Perhaps a lasting revolution in sex education will not be based on who the audience is, but rather the form the education takes. The Internet, for all its limits, can provide factual, empowering information, if only people can sift the fact from the fiction. Perhaps to do that, a whole new understanding of expertise must take root. And that, of course, might be a long revolution.

Notes

Introduction

1. J. W. Gibson, Mrs. J. W. Gibson, and W. J. Truitt, *Golden Thoughts on Chastity and Procreation* (Naperville, IL: J. L. Nichols, 1903), 258.

2. J. W. Gibson, Mrs. J. W. Gibson, and W. J. Truitt, *Social Purity, or, the Life of the Home and Nation* (Naperville, IL: J. L. Nichols, 1903).

3. "The Two Paths" (illustration from *Social Purity, or, the Life of the Home and Nation*, 1903), Library of Congress, American Women: The General Collections. HQ31.G46, accessed April 15, 2006. http://memory.loc.gov/ammem/awhhtml/ awgc1/d18.html.

4. Michele Mitchell theorizes that the text was originally written for white audiences. At least one author, John Gibson, is inconsistently described to be white in historical records. See Mitchell, *Righteous Propagation: African Americans and the Politics of Racial Destiny after Reconstruction* (Chapel Hill: University of North Carolina Press, 2004), 87–90.

5. The term "middle class" does not necessarily carry the same meaning for whites and blacks in the early twentieth century. While the white middle class could be defined economically, the black middle class (or aspiring class) could be defined by education and "respectability" rather than wealth. Additionally, only those with disposable income and access to education would have been consumers of advice literature.

6. For more on normalization, see Julian B. Carter, *The Heart of Whiteness: Normal Sexuality and Race in America, 1880–1940* (Durham: Duke University Press, 2007), chapter 3.

7. For an overview of the historical construction of sexuality, see Michel Foucault, *The History of Sexuality*, vol. 1, *An Introduction* (New York, Pantheon Books, 1976); John D'Emilio and Estelle Freedman, *Intimate Matters: A History of Sexuality in America* (New York: Harper and Row, 1988); Martin Bauml Duberman, Martha Vicinus, and George Chauncey Jr., *Hidden from History: Reclaiming the Gay and Lesbian Past* (New York: New American Library, 1989).

8. See, for example, Wallace Maw, "Fifty Years of Sex Education in the Public Schools of the United States (1900–1950): A History of Ideas" (PhD diss., University of Cincinnati, 1953); James R. Cook, "The Evolution of Sex Education in the Public Schools of the United States, 1900–1970" (PhD diss., Southern Illinois University, 1971); David Pivar, *Purity Crusade: Sexuality, Morality, and Social Control, 1868–1900* (Westport, CT: Greenwood Press, 1973). John C. Burnham, "The Progressive Era Revolution in American Attitudes toward Sex," *Journal of American History* 59,

no. 4 (1973): 885–908. Ronald G. Walters, *Primers for Prudery: Sexual Advice to Victorian America* (Englewood Cliffs, NJ: Prentice-Hall, 1973); Michael Imber, "Analysis of a Curriculum Reform Movement: The American Social Hygiene Association's Campaign for Sex Education, 1900–1930" (PhD diss., Stanford University, 1980); Patricia J. Campbell, *Sex Guides: Books and Films about Sexuality for Young Adults* (New York: Garland, 1986); Michael Edward Melody and Linda Mary Peterson, *Teaching America about Sex: Marriage Guides and Sex Manuals from the Late Victorians to Dr. Ruth* (New York: New York University Press, 1999); Jeffrey P. Moran, *Teaching Sex: The Shaping of Adolescence in the Twentieth Century* (Cambridge, MA: Harvard University Press, 2000).

9. For recent work on the links among eugenics, immigration, and sexuality, see Margot Canaday, *The Straight State: Sexuality and Citizenship in Twentieth-Century America* (Princeton, NJ: Princeton University Press, 2009); and Alexandra Minna Stern, *Eugenic Nation: Faults and Frontiers of Better Breeding in Modern America* (Berkeley, University of California Press, 2005).

10. Nancy K. Bristow, *Making Men Moral: Social Engineering during the Great War* (New York: New York University Press, 1996); Alexandra M. Lord, *Condom Nation: The U.S. Government's Sex Education Campaign from World War I to the Internet.* Baltimore: Johns Hopkins University Press, 2009. For an analysis of issues of national identity, patriotism, and sexuality in Canada, see Christabelle Sethna, "The Facts of Life: The Sex Instruction of Ontario Public School Children, 1900–1950" (PhD diss., University of Toronto, 1995).

11. Jennifer Burek Pierce, *What Adolescents Ought to Know: Sexual Health Texts in Early Twentieth-Century America* (Amherst: University of Massachusetts Press, 2011). Pierce draws the work of Roy Porter and Lesley Hall on European sex education literature. See Porter and Hall, *The Facts of Life: The Creation of Sexual Knowledge in Britain* (New Haven, CT: Yale University Press, 1995).

12. Robert Eberwein, *Sex Ed: Film, Video, and the Framework of Desire* (New Brunswick, NJ: Rutgers University Press, 1999); Sharon R. Ullman, *Sex Seen: The Emergence of Modern Sexuality in America* (Berkeley: University of California Press, 1997); Martin Pernick, *The Black Stork: Eugenics and the Death of "Defective" Babies in American Medicine and Motion Pictures since 1915* (New York: Oxford University Press, 1996). The use of alternative media, be they visual presentations or radio shows, influenced the ways audiences received and interpreted the material. See also Alison Bashford and Carolyn Strange, "Public Pedagogy: Sex Education and Mass Communication in the Mid-twentieth Century," *Journal of the History of Sexuality* 13, no. 1 (2004): 71–99.

13. Jessamyn Neuhaus, "The Importance of Being Orgasmic: Sexuality, Gender, and Marital Sex Manuals in the United States, 1920–1963," *Journal of the History of Sexuality* 9, no. 4 (2000): 447–73; Susan K. Freeman, *Sex Goes to School: Girls and Sex Education before the 1960s* (Urbana: University of Illinois Press, 2008).

14. Leigh Ann Wheeler, "Rescuing Sex from Prudery and Prurience: American Women's Use of Sex Education as an Antidote to Obscenity, 1925–1932," *Journal of Women's History* 12, no. 3 (2000): 173–95.

15. I use Nancy Cott's term, "passionlessness," here to denote the so-called Victorian assumption that women lacked sexual desire or agency. See Nancy Cott, "Passionlessness: An Interpretation of Victorian Sexual Ideology, 1790–1850," *Signs:*

Journal of Women in Culture and Society 4, no. 2 (1978): 219–36. On black women's use of (and exploitation by) the sexual marketplace, see Erin D. Chapman, *Prove It on Me: New Negroes, Sex, and Popular Culture in the 1920s* (New York: Oxford University Press, 2012), chapter 3.

16. Alexandra M. Lord, "Models of Masculinity: Sex Education, the United States Public Health Service, and the YMCA, 1919–1924," *Journal of the History of Medicine and Allied Sciences* 58, no. 2 (2003): 123–52; Alexandra M. Lord, "'Naturally Clean and Wholesome': Women, Sex Education, and the United States Public Health Service, 1918–1928," *Social History of Medicine* 17, no. 3 (2004): 423–41.

Chapter One

1. Denslow Lewis, *The Gynecologic Consideration of the Sexual Act* (Chicago: Henry O. Shepard, 1900), 20–23.

2. Delcevare King to Prince A. Morrow, May 23, 1910, folder 1:1, ASHA Papers.

3. Prince A. Morrow to Delcevare King, May 24, 1910, folder 1:1, ASHA Papers.

4. Prince A. Morrow to Mrs. John Storer Cobb, April 13, 1909, folder 1:4, ASHA Papers.

5. Historically, those labeled "sex radicals" either had or were assumed to have politically and socially radical beliefs as well. See Christine Stansell, *American Moderns: Bohemian New York and the Creation of a New Century* (New York: Metropolitan Books, 2000).

6. Maurice A. Bigelow, *Sex-Education: A Series of Lectures Concerning the Knowledge of Sex in Its Relation to Human Life* (New York: Macmillan, 1916), 11.

7. Amanda Frisken, *Victoria Woodhull's Sexual Revolution: Political Theater and the Popular Press in Nineteenth-Century America* (Philadelphia: University of Pennsylvania Press, 2004).

8. This contradiction is at the heart of Jennifer Burek Pierce's work on sex hygiene texts in print culture. See Pierce, *What Adolescents Ought to Know*, 184.

9. Ibid., 35. Attempts to limit access to sexual information has long been a tradition in the sex education movement. See Martha Cornog, *For Sex Education, See Librarian: A Guide to Issues and Resources* (New York: Greenwood Press, 1996), chapter 2.

10. Margaret Sanger, *Margaret Sanger: An Autobiography* (New York: W. W. Norton, 1938), 93–94; Jean H. Baker, *Margaret Sanger: A Life of Passion* (New York: Hill and Wang, 2011), 72. Sanger claimed to have consulted major libraries such as the Academy of Medicine, the Library of Congress, and the Boston Public Library. This may have been part of the problem, as popular literature may not have found its way into libraries but could be purchased through newspaper advertisements.

11. Baker, *Margaret Sanger*, 56–62.

12. Ellen Chesler, *Woman of Valor: Margaret Sanger and the Birth Control Movement in America* (New York: Simon and Schuster, 1992), 65–66.

13. Some of the best known were Robert Dale Owen, *Moral Physiology, or a Brief and Plain Treatise on the Population Question* (New York: G. Vale, 1830); Charles Knowlton, *Fruits of Philosophy, or the Private Companion of Adult People* (Philadelphia:

F. P. Rogers, 1839); Alice B. Stockham, *Tokology: A Book for Every Woman*, 1894 ed. (Chicago: Alice B. Stockham, 1887).

14. A major problem with the study of sexual behavior and beliefs is evidentiary: the nineteenth century encompasses a time of increased privacy within marriage, so state intervention (and thus evidence of sexual behavior) in sexual matters decreased. Historians have turned from court cases to advice literature, popular culture, and personal documents like letters and diaries to gather evidence.

15. Estelle Freedman, "Sexuality in Nineteenth-Century America: Behavior, Ideology, and Politics," *Reviews in American History* 10 (December 1982): 201; John S. Haller and Robin M. Haller, *The Physician and Sexuality in Victorian America*, rev. ed. (Carbondale: Southern Illinois University Press, 1995), chapter 3.

16. Burnham, "Progressive Era Revolution," 881.

17. Melody and Peterson, *Teaching America about Sex*, chapter 1.

18. Mark Thomas Connelly, *The Response to Prostitution in the Progressive Era* (Chapel Hill: University of North Carolina Press, 1980), 8–9.

19. Walters, *Primers for Prudery*. For more on alternate ideas about marriage and sexuality in the nineteenth century, see Robert David Thomas, *The Man Who Would Be Perfect: John Humphrey Noyes and the Utopian Impulse* (Philadelphia: University of Pennsylvania Press, 1977); Louis Kern, *An Ordered Love: Sex Roles and Sexuality in Victorian Utopias: The Shakers, the Mormons, and the Oneida Community* (Chapel Hill: University of North Carolina Press, 1981); John C. Spurlock, *Free Love: Marriage and Middle-Class Radicalism in America, 1825–1860* (New York: New York University Press, 1988).

20. Burnham, "Progressive Era Revolution."

21. Ibid., 885.

22. Bigelow, *Sex-Education*, 12.

23. Ibid., 14.

24. Pivar, *Purity Crusade*, chapter 1.

25. B. E. De Costa, "The White Cross Movement," *Philanthropist* 1, no. 1 (1886): 1.

26. Ibid.

27. Pivar, *Purity Crusade*, 112–14.

28. For the construction of cultural whiteness, see Matthew Frye Jacobson, *Whiteness of a Different Color: European Immigrants and the Alchemy of Race* (Cambridge, MA: Harvard University Press, 1998); David Roediger, *The Wages of Whiteness: Race and the Making of the American Working Class* (London: Verso, 1991). For a discussion of the construction of sexual whiteness, see Carter, *Heart of Whiteness*, introduction.

29. See especially Frances E. Willard, "Frances E. Willard on Social Purity," *Philanthropist* 1, no. 1 (1886): 2.

30. "Legal Protection for Young Girls," *Philanthropist* 1, no. 1 (1886): 4–5.

31. Some purity advocates were beginning to call into question the nineteenth century belief that poverty resulted from moral failing, be it intemperance or promiscuity. See William Lloyd Garrison, "The Relation of Poverty to Purity," in *The National Purity Congress*, ed. Aaron M. Powell (New York: American Purity Alliance, 1896), 398–405.

32. Anna Rice Powell, "The Moral Elevation of Girls," *Philanthropist* 1, no. 2 (1886): 3.

33. Aaron M. Powell, ed., *The National Purity Congress: Its Papers, Addresses, Portraits* (New York: American Purity Alliance, 1896), 174–78.

34. Ibid., 328.

35. For more on Frances E. W. Harper, see Alison M. Parker, *Articulating Rights: Nineteenth-Century American Women on Race, Reform, and the State* (DeKalb: Northern Illinois Press, 2010), chapter 3.

36. "Medical Declaration Concerning Chastity," *Philanthropist* 10, no. 1 (1895): 5. Powell included periodic updates of the list, including the names of the physicians who had signed the declaration and additional editorial comments the physicians added. See the May 1895 issue.

37. Walter Clarke, "Dr. Prince Albert Morrow and His Aides," *Journal of Social Hygiene* 40, no. 5 (1954): 181.

38. Prince A. Morrow, "The Prophylaxis of Venereal Diseases: Medical Aspects of the Social Evil in New York," *Philadelphia Medical Journal* 7 (1901): 667. The interaction between these two factions is the subject of David Pivar, *Purity and Hygiene: Women, Prostitution, and the "American Plan," 1900–1930* (Westport, CT: Greenwood Press, 2002).

39. Burnham, "Progressive Era Revolution," 897–98.

40. Ibid., 900.

41. Prince A. Morrow, *Social Diseases and Marriage* (New York: Lea Brothers, 1904), 348. This was a common tactic for medical professionals, who noted the dangers of disease since germs do not obey the same sorts of social (or racial) stratification that people might. Morrow used the specter of class mixing to denote the fear that lower-class diseases could threaten the middle class. See chapter 4 for more on racial segregation and venereal disease.

42. Ibid.; Morrow, "Prophylaxis of Venereal Diseases," 665; Allan M. Brandt, *No Magic Bullet: A Social History of Venereal Disease in the United States since 1880* (New York: Oxford University Press, 1985). For a cross-national analysis of gender and venereal disease treatment, see Jill Harsin, "Syphilis, Wives, and Physicians: Medical Ethics and the Family in Late Nineteenth-Century Paris," *French Historical Studies* 16, no. 1 (1989): 72–95.

43. Morrow, *Social Diseases and Marriage*, 348–49.

44. Ibid., 352.

45. The late nineteenth and early twentieth centuries witnessed expanded educational opportunities for women, especially in the sciences. Yet it was still expected that scientific training would lead not to equal opportunity but to providing women the skills necessary to better fulfill their proper gender roles as wives, mothers, and helpers. Ultimate subordination to male scientific authority remained. See Rima D. Apple, *Mothers and Medicine: A Social History of Infant Feeding, 1890–1950* (Madison: University of Wisconsin Press, 1987), part 3; Margaret W. Rossiter, *Women Scientists in America*, vol. 1, *Struggles and Strategies to 1940* (Baltimore: Johns Hopkins University Press, 1982), chapter 3.

46. Morrow, *Social Diseases and Marriage*, 360.

47. Moran, *Teaching Sex*, 23–28.

48. William F. Snow, "Progress: 1900–1915," in *American Social Hygiene Association* (Minneapolis: 1915), 40–41.

49. E. L. Keyes, "Personals," *Survey*, April 12, 1913, 76.

50. Prince A. Morrow, *Publicity as a Factor in Venereal Prophylaxis* (Chicago: Press of the American Medical Association, 1906), 2.

51. For an overview on muckraking and Progressivism, see the work of Louis Filler, especially *Muckraking and Progressivism in the American Tradition* (New Brunswick, NJ: Transaction Press, 1996).

52. Morrow, *Publicity as a Factor in Venereal Prophylaxis*, 7.

53. Ibid., 6.

54. Morrow, "Prophylaxis of Venereal Diseases," 664.

55. Ibid., 663.

56. Pierce, *What Adolescents Ought to Know*, chapter 3. Indiana was the first of many states to pass eugenic sterilization laws. See Philip Reilly, *The Surgical Solution: A History of Involuntary Sterilization in the United States* (Baltimore: Johns Hopkins University Press, 1991).

57. St. Louis proved a fertile ground for the purity movement, since it was the site of the nation's first experiment with regulated prostitution in the 1870s.

58. For an excellent discussion of the relation between the purity and hygiene wings of the movement, see Pivar, *Purity and Hygiene.*

59. Jason Bronson Reynolds, "The Union of the American Vigilance Association and the American Federation for Sex Hygiene," *Vigilance* 27, no. 10 (1913): 1.

60. Morrow, *Social Diseases and Marriage*, 363.

61. *First Annual Report, 1913–1914*, October 9, 1914, 4–6, ASHA Papers.

62. Ibid.

63. Morrow, "Prophylaxis of Venereal Diseases," 663.

64. *First Annual Report, 1913–1914*, 12, 19.

65. "Recommendations as to Work of the Law Department of the American Social Hygiene Association," February 13, 1914, folder 5:2, ASHA Papers; "Prospects in the South," *American Social Hygiene Association Bulletin* 1, no. 3 (1914): 1. Some local organizations took the initiative without ties to the national organization. For example, Dr. Malone Duggan of San Antonio, Texas, published sex education articles in the *Texas Medical Journal* and *Texas State Journal of Medicine* as early as 1909 and worked extensively with area women's clubs.

66. See, for example, David Arnold, *Colonizing the Body: State Medicine and Epidemic Disease in Nineteenth-Century India* (Berkeley: University of California Press, 1993); Mark Harrison, "The Tender Frame of Man: Disease, Climate, and Racial Difference in India and the West Indies, 1760–1860," *Bulletin of the History of Medicine* 70, no. 1 (1996): 68–93; Alexander Butchart, *The Anatomy of Power: European Constructions of the African Body* (London: Zed Books, 1998).

67. Stern, *Eugenic Nation*, 28.

68. Minutes, Executive Committee Meeting, March 12, 1914, folder 5:2, ASHA Papers.

69. *Second Annual Report, 1914–1915*, October 8, 1915, 7–8, folder 19:5, ASHA Papers.

70. Thomas D. Eliot, "Social Hygiene at the Panama-Pacific International Exposition," *Journal of Social Hygiene* 1, no. 3 (1915): 398.

71. Ibid., 413.

72. Stern, *Eugenic Nation*, 34; Natalia Molina, *Fit to Be Citizens? Public Health and Race in Los Angeles, 1879–1939* (Berkeley: University of California Press, 2006):

26–29. California maintained a high level of interest in racial health and eugenics. The state led the nation in eugenic sterilizations.

73. Ibid., 408.

74. Florence Crittenden Leagues provided homes, support, and adoption services to unwed mothers.

75. Stern, *Eugenic Nation*, chapter 1.

Chapter Two

1. Robert Willson, "An Outline Program for the Teaching of Sex Hygiene in the Schools," in *Transactions of the Fourth International Congress on School Hygiene*, 3:29.

2. Lawrence Cremin, *The Transformation of the School: Progressivism in American Education, 1876–1957* (New York: Alfred A. Knopf, 1961), 71. See all of chapter 3 for a full discussion of the expansion of school responsibilities in the community.

3. Ibid., 171. Americanization tended to take the form of Anglicization, with well-documented efforts by schools to disrupt foreign language and cultural practices, encourage patriotism, and discourage political and economic radicalism. See, for example, Mary Antin, *The Promised Land* (Boston: Houghton Mifflin, 1912); John Higham, *Strangers in the Land: Patterns of American Nativism, 1860–1925* (New Brunswick, NJ: Rutgers University Press, 1955).

4. Cremin, *Transformation of the School*, 17–18.

5. Charles W. Eliot, *The Training for an Effective Life* (Boston: Houghton Mifflin, 1915), 74–75.

6. Charles W. Eliot, "The American Social Hygiene Association," *Social Hygiene* 1, no. 1 (1914): 2.

7. Quoted in Snow, "Progress."

8. See, for example, Glenda Elizabeth Gilmore, *Gender and Jim Crow: Women and the Politics of White Supremacy in North Carolina, 1896–1920* (Chapel Hill: University of North Carolina Press, 1996), 31–37; Peter Irons, *Jim Crow's Children: The Broken Promise of the Brown Decision* (New York: Viking Penguin, 2002): chapters 1–2.

9. James D. Phelan, "The Japanese Evil in California," *North American Review* 21, no. 762 (September 1919): 325.

10. Cremin, *Transformation of the School*, 3–8.

11. David Tyack and Larry Cuban, *Tinkering toward Utopia: A Century of Public School Reform* (Cambridge, MA: Harvard University Press, 1995), 47–48.

12. Cremin, *Transformation of the School*, 93.

13. For example, the Rockefeller Foundation's General Education Fund stipulated industrial and vocational training programs for African American students. See John Ensor Harr and Peter J. Johnson, *The Rockefeller Century* (New York: Scribner's, 1988), 70–82.

14. Paul E. Peterson, *The Politics of School Reform, 1870–1940* (Chicago: University of Chicago Press, 1985), chapter 5; Elisabeth Lasch-Quinn, *Black Neighbors: Race and the Limits of Reform in the American Settlement House Movement, 1890–1945* (Chapel Hill: University of North Carolina Press, 1993).

15. ASHA's work would not come to fruition until the 1920s, when a significant minority of schools adopted at least some sex education into their

curriculum. Michael Imber's analysis of the nature of curriculum reform, and the importance of shaping the debate, notes how the early failures made later successes possible. See Imber, "Toward a Theory of Curriculum Reform: An Analysis of the First Campaign for Sex Education," *Curriculum Inquiry* 12, no. 4 (1982): 339–62. For a more generalized discussion of the power of the debate over free love and the eventual "sexual revolution" of the 1920s, see Stansell, *American Moderns*, chapter 8.

16. Cremin, *Transformation of the School*, 168–69.

17. Imber, "Toward a Theory of Curriculum Reform," 348.

18. Bigelow, *Sex-Education*, vii, 108.

19. Imber, "Toward a Theory of Curriculum Reform," 353–54.

20. William Robinson to Mary S. Cobb, December 7, 1910, folder 1:4, ASHA Papers.

21. William J. Robinson, *Sex Knowledge for Men Including a Program for Sex Education of the Boy* (New York: Critic and Guide, 1916), 1, 244.

22. Stansell, *American Moderns*, chapter 8; Margaret Sanger, "No Gods No Masters," *Woman Rebel* 1, no. 1 (1914): 1, 8, 16.

23. "Teaching Sex Knowledge," *Boston Traveler*, 1915, folder 1:3, ASHA Papers.

24. Imber, "Toward a Theory of Curriculum Reform," 349, 351.

25. Richard H. Tierney, "The Catholic Church and the Sex Problem," *Journal of Education*, September 25, 1913, 285–86.

26. "The New Game of Playing with Fire and the Right Not to Be Forced to Know Evil," *Century*, March 1913, 796.

27. "Letters of May 1912," May 1, 1914, folder 170:9, ASHA Papers.

28. Quoted in Imber, "Toward a Theory of Curriculum Reform," 354.

29. Peterson, *Politics of School Reform*, 110.

30. Molina, *Fit to Be Citizens*, chapter 2.

31. Robert Wiebe, *The Search for Order, 1877–1920* (New York: Hill and Wang, 1967), 57–58.

32. "Letters of May 1912," 1 May 1914, folder 170:9, ASHA Papers.

33. "Some Propositions concerning Teaching Sex Hygiene," June 3, 1912, folder L1:1, ASHA Papers.

34. Steven Mintz, *Huck's Raft: A History of American Childhood* (Cambridge, MA: Belknap Press, 2004), chapter 7.

35. I use the term to describe those states with a heritage of slavery and secession. These states developed a peculiar racial legal and social system by the turn of the twentieth century, including Jim Crow legislation and a resistance to federal interference due to the legacy of Reconstruction. See Edward L. Ayers, *The Promise of the New South: Life after Reconstruction* (New York: Oxford University Press, 1992), 3–4; C. Vann Woodward, *The Burden of Southern History* (Baton Rouge: Louisiana State University Press, 1960), 3–25; C. Vann Woodward, *Origins of the New South, 1877–1913* (Baton Rouge: Louisiana State University, 1951), preface.

36. Lawrence Cremin, *American Education: The Metropolitan Experience, 1876–1980* (New York: Harper and Row, 1988).

37. Pamela Barnhouse Walters and Philip J. O'Connell, "The Family Economy, Work, and Educational Participation in the United States, 1890–1940," *American Journal of Sociology* 93, no. 5 (1988): 116–52.

38. Peterson, *Politics of School Reform*, 52–60. This was especially true of segregated schools in the South.

39. John Ettling, *The Germ of Laziness: Rockefeller Philanthropy and Public Health in the New South* (Cambridge, MA: Harvard University Press, 1981); Elizabeth W. Etheridge, *The Butterfly Caste: A Social History of Pellagra in the South* (Westport, CT: Greenwood Press, 1972).

40. Jeffrey P. Moran, "'Modernism Gone Mad': Sex Education Comes to Chicago, 1913," *Journal of American History* 83, no. 2 (1996): 500–502.

41. Imber, "Toward a Theory of Curriculum Reform"; Lavinia Dock, *Hygiene and Morality: A Manual for Nurses and Others, Giving an Outline of the Medical, Social, and Legal Aspects of Venereal Diseases* (New York: G. P. Putnam's Sons, 1910).

42. Wiebe, *Search for Order*, 157.

43. Moran, *Teaching Sex*, 53; Imber, "Toward a Theory of Curriculum Reform." 356.

44. Moran, "Modernism Gone Mad," 502.

45. Ibid., 508.

46. Moran, *Teaching Sex*, 55–58.

47. Jonathan Zimmerman, *Distilling Democracy: Alcohol Education in America's Public Schools, 1880–1925* (Lawrence: University Press of Kansas, 1999), chapter 2.

48. Imber, "Analysis of a Curriculum Reform Movement," 30–31; Carl F. Kaestle, *Pillars of the Republic: Common Schools and American Society 1780–1860* (New York: Hill and Wang, 1983).

49. "Some Propositions concerning Teaching Sex Hygiene."

50. "Bars out Sex Hygiene," *New York Times*, October 26, 1913.

51. "Sex Topics in the Schools," *Journal of Education*, November 27, 1913, 538.

52. Committee of Education, minutes, January 13, 1912, folder 3:6, ASHA Papers.

53. "Letters of May 1912," May 1, 1914, folder 170:9, ASHA Papers.

54. Eliot, "Social Hygiene at the Panama-Pacific International Exposition," 403.

55. Ibid., 405.

56. Edward Howard Griggs, *Moral Education* (Croton-on-Hudson: Orchard Hill Press, 1903), 269.

57. Ibid., 270.

58. Edward Lyttleton, "Instructions in Matters of Sex," *Educational Review* 46 (1913): 137–38.

59. Ibid., 141.

60. Ibid., 142.

61. Prince A. Morrow to Mary S. Cobb, October 30, 1909, folder 1:4, ASHA Papers.

62. "Letters of May 1912," May 1, 1914, folder 170:9, ASHA Papers.

63. *First Annual Report, 1913–1914*, 9 October 1914, p. 6, folder 19:5, ASHA Papers.

Chapter Three

1. James Jones, *Alfred C. Kinsey: A Life* (New York: W. W. Norton, 1997), 74–75.

2. For more on the purported crisis of masculinity, see Peter G. Filene, *Him/Her/Self: Sex Roles in Modern America* (New York: Harcourt Brace Jovanovich, 1975); E. Anthony Rotundo, *American Manhood: Transformations in Masculinity from the Revolution to the Modern Era* (New York: Basic Books, 1993).

3. Thomas G. Dyer, *Theodore Roosevelt and the Idea of Race* (Baton Rouge: Louisiana State University Press, 1980); Theodore Roosevelt, *The Strenuous Life: Essays and Addresses* (New York: Century, 1901).

4. See, for example, Maw, "Fifty Years of Sex Education"; Cook, "Evolution of Sex Education"; Imber, "Analysis of a Curriculum Reform Movement."

5. Moran, *Teaching Sex.* For a criticism of Moran's work, see Lori Rotskoff, "Sex in the Schools: Adolescence, Sex Education, and Social Reform," *Reviews in American History* 29, no. 2 (2001): 310–18.

6. Joseph F. Kett, *Rites of Passage: Adolescence in America, 1790 to the Present* (New York: Basic Books, 1977).

7. Hall was himself a product of the northeastern white middle class. Hall's construction of adolescence also excluded much of girls' experience, since girls did not have the same schooling and career options available to boys of the same class and race, although this was changing rapidly. See also Jane H. Hunter, *How Young Ladies Became Girls: The Victorian Origins of American Girlhood* (New Haven, CT: Yale University Press, 2002).

8. See Herbert Gutman, *The Black Family in Slavery and Freedom, 1750–1925* (New York: Vintage Books, 1976), chapter 10; Mintz, *Huck's Raft*, chapter 7. These works also illustrate how region played a critical role in educational opportunity, with urban and suburban northeasterners having more access to high schools than did rural, western, and southern adolescents.

9. Kett, *Rites of Passage*, 190.

10. Recapitulation was first introduced by biologist Ernst Haeckel, who applied it to embryological development. G. Stanley Hall then applied it to childhood. See Ernst Haeckel, *The Riddle of the Universe at the Close of the Nineteenth Century*, trans. Joseph McCabe (New York: Harper, 1900); G. Stanley Hall, *Adolescence: Its Psychology and Its Relations to Physiology, Anthropology, Sociology, Sex, Crime, Religion, and Education* (New York: Appleton, 1904); Gail Bederman, *Manliness and Civilization: A Cultural History of Gender and Race in the United States, 1880–1917* (Chicago: University of Chicago Press, 1995), chapter 3.

11. William Byron Forbush, *The Boy Problem: A Study in Social Pedagogy* (Boston: Pilgrim Press, 1901), 23, 148. The Boy Scouts of America fully embraced Hall's theories, including in *The Scout Master's Handbook* an extensive discussion of recapitulation theory. See BSA, *Handbook for Scout Masters, Boy Scouts of America* (New York: BSA, 1914), 94–96. For a discussion of Forbush's popularity, see Robert H. MacDonald, *Sons of the Empire: The Frontier and the Boy Scout Movement* (Toronto: University of Toronto Press, 1993), 141.

12. Forbush, *Boy Problem*, 29–31.

13. Clelia Duel Mosher, *The Mosher Survey: Sexual Attitudes of 45 Victorian Women* (New York: Arno Press, 1980). Mosher performed her research between 1892 and 1920, although her results were not published until 1980.

14. Katherine Bement Davis, *Factors in the Sex Life of Twenty-Two Hundred Women* (New York: Harper & Brothers, 1929). For more mentions of the Bible as a sex education text, see Mosher, *Mosher Survey*, 325, 42, 67, 90.

NOTES TO PP. 34–38 159

15. Davis, *Factors in the Sex Life of Twenty-Two Hundred Women.* Home remedy books often included incomplete information about puberty and reproduction that raised more questions than they answered. *The Cottage Physician*, for instance, has a chapter on menstruation without discussing the mechanics of blood loss. George W. Post, *The Cottage Physician: For Individual and Family Use* (Springfield: King-Richardson, 1897), 267–69.

16. While this was not universally true, and most likely poorly enforced, many medical texts, especially those specializing in sexual health, carried a warning that they were intended only for the medical profession. Warnings such as these, however, may have actually increased lay demand for such books. See Walter Franklin Robie, *Sex Histories: Authentic Sex Experiences of Men and Women Showing How Fear and Ignorance of the Sex Life Lead to Individual Misery and Social Depravity* (London: Amalgamated Medical Press, 1922).

17. Hall, *Adolescence*, 1:437.

18. Ibid., 1:452. Hall did not actively support Cohn's suggestion, but he did not entirely dismiss it either.

19. Some evangelical Christian authors have recently reemphasized the importance of the Bible as the best, if not only, source for sex education. See Amy DeRogatis, "What Would Jesus Do? Sexuality and Salvation in Protestant Evangelical Sex Manuals, 1950s to the Present," *Church History* 74, no. 1 (2005): 97–137.

20. "Plain Sex Truths Are Told by Daddy to Men and Women," *San Antonio Express*, November 16, 1917, 4.

21. Kett, *Rites of Passage*, 199–200.

22. George J. Fisher, "Sex Education in the Young Men's Christian Association," *Journal of Social Hygiene* 1, no. 2 (1915): 230; Bigelow, *Sex-Education*, 156.

23. Nina Mjagkij, *Light in the Darkness: African Americans and the YMCA 1852–1946* (Lexington: University of Kentucky Press, 1994), 1–2, 25–26.

24. Fisher, "Sex Education in the Young Men's Christian Association," 226.

25. Ibid., 230.

26. M. J. Exner, "Sex Education Literature for Boys and Men," *American Youth* 2, no. 1 (1913): 74.

27. Ibid., 75.

28. Bigelow, *Sex-Education*, 51, 122–23.

29. Mjagkij, *Light in the Darkness*, 33.

30. Exner, "Sex Education Literature for Boys and Men," 80.

31. Aaron G. Knebel, *Four Decades with Men and Boys* (New York: Association Press, 1936), 14.

32. Ibid., 84.

33. Ibid., 85.

34. Ibid., 86. For more on the protection of white male sexual prerogative, see Leslie K. Dunlap, "The Reform of Rape Law and the Problem of White Men: Age-of-Consent Campaigns in the South, 1885–1910," in *Sex, Love, Race: Crossing Boundaries in North American History*, ed. Martha Hodes (New York: New York University Press, 1999), 352–72.

35. A. H. Finn, "Detroit Sex Hygiene Campaign," *Survey*, December 17, 1910, 460–61.

36. Winfield Scott Hall, *The Biology, Physiology and Sociology of Reproduction, Also Sexual Hygiene, with Special Reference to the Male* (Chicago: Wynnewood, 1907), 150–51.

37. For example, the YMCA of Greater San Antonio today takes as its mission "to put Judeo-Christian principles into practice though programs that build a healthy spirit, mind and body for all." YMCA of Greater San Antonio, "Christian Heritage," accessed August 8, 2014. http://www.ymcasatx.org/page.aspx?pid=2151.

38. Eli Lederhendler, *Jewish Responses to Modernity: New Voices in America and Eastern Europe* (New York: New York University Press, 1994), 111.

39. Chesler, *Woman of Valor*, 150–51.

40. Lederhendler, *Jewish Responses*, 144.

41. Ibid., 146.

42. Emma Goldman, *Living My Life* (New York: Alfred A. Knopf, 1931), chapter 45; Baker, *Margaret Sanger*, 170.

43. Lederhendler, *Jewish Responses*, 148–52.

44. Ibid., 158.

45. David I. Macleod, *Building Character in the American Boy: The Boy Scouts, YMCA, and Their Forerunners, 1870–1920* (Madison: University of Wisconsin Press, 1983), 213.

46. Ibid., 17, 37, 97.

47. BSA, *Handbook for Scout Masters*, 72–73.

48. Hall, *Adolescence*, 325–33.

49. Macleod, *Building Character*, 213.

50. BSA, *Handbook for Scout Masters*, 74. Emphasis in original.

51. Ibid., 90.

52. Ibid., 94. This is a reference to masturbation.

53. Ibid., 108.

54. Macleod, *Building Character*, 300.

55. Luther Gulick, "Boys' and Girls' Organizations and Social Hygiene," *Journal of the Society of Sanitary and Moral Prophylaxis* 5 (1914): 192.

56. BSA, *The Official Handbook for Boys* (New York: Doubleday: 1913), 520–21.

57. Jay Mechling, *On My Honor: Boy Scouts and the Making of American Youth* (Chicago: University of Chicago Press, 2001). Mechling's anthropological study of Boy Scout members bridges the gap between the ideology of the organization and the ways in which boys experienced scouting.

58. "Sex Hygiene Lectures Given to Boy Scouts," *Scouting* 1, no. 10 (1913): 8.

59. Macleod, *Building Character*, 260.

60. Mjagkij, *Light in the Darkness*, chapter 3.

61. Macleod, *Building Character*, 197.

62. H. Paul Douglass, *How Shall the Country Youth Be Served? A Study of "Rural" Work of Certain Character-Building Agencies* (New York: George H. Doran, 1926), 162.

63. Clark W. Hetherington, "Play Leadership in Sex Education," *Journal of Social Hygiene* 1, no. 1 (1914): 37.

64. Ibid., 41.

65. Hall, *Adolescence*, 1:472–512.

66. Constance A. Nathanson, *Dangerous Passage: The Social Control of Sexuality in Women's Adolescence* (Philadelphia: Temple University Press, 1991), 77; Hunter, *How Young Ladies Became Girls*, chapters 7 and 9.

67. Hall, *Adolescence*, vol. 2, chapter 17. See also Edward Clarke, *Sex in Education, or a Fair Chance for Girls* (Boston: Harvard University Press, 1873); and Lisa Carstens, "Unbecoming Women: Sex Reversal in the Scientific Discourse on Female Deviance in Britain, 1880–1920, *Journal of the History of Sexuality* 20, no. 1 (2011): 62–95.

68. Joan Jacobs Brumberg, "'Something Happens to Girls': Menarche and the Emergence of the Modern American Hygiene Imperative," *Journal of the History of Sexuality* 4, no. 1 (1993): 99–127.

69. The link is attributable to better nutrition available to girls of the upper classes. See Elizabeth Blackwell, *The Laws of Life with Special Reference to the Physical Education of Girls* (New York: G. P. Putnam, 1852).

70. Carroll Smith-Rosenberg and Charles Rosenberg, "The Female Animal: Medical and Biological Views of Woman and Her Role in Nineteenth-Century America," *Journal of American History* 60, no. 2 (1973): 338–41; Mel Davies, "Corsets and Conception: Fashion and Demographic Trends in the Nineteenth Century," *Comparative Studies in Society and History* 24, no. 4 (1982): 631–32. For more on the connection among race, physiology, and sexual precocity, see Sander L. Gilman, *Difference and Pathology: Stereotypes of Sexuality, Race, and Madness* (Ithaca, NY: Cornell University Press, 1985), 98.

71. Hall, *Adolescence*, 1:474–76.

72. Carroll Smith-Rosenberg, *Disorderly Conduct: Visions of Gender in Victorian America* (New York: Alfred A. Knopf, 1985), chapter 8.

73. Thomas Faulkner and J. H. Carmichael, *The Cottage Physician: Best Known Methods of Treatment in All Diseases, Accidents and Emergencies of the Home* (Springfield, MA: King, Richardson, 1892), 546.

74. Joan Jacobs Brumberg, *The Body Project: An Intimate History of American Girls* (New York: Random House, 1997), 10.

75. Hunter, *How Young Ladies Became Girls*, chapter 5.

76. For an example of physicians interjecting themselves in traditionally women's practices such as infant feeding, see Apple, *Mothers and Medicine*.

77. Brumberg, *The Body Project*, 34.

78. Pierce, *What Adolescents Ought to Know*, 35.

79. Winfield Scott Hall, *Daughter, Mother and Father: A Story for Girls* (Chicago: AMA Press, 1913).

80. Brumberg, *Body Project*, chapter 2.

81. For more on passionlessness, see Barbara Welter, "The Cult of True Womanhood, 1820–1860," *American Quarterly* 18, no. 2 (1966): 151–74; Nancy Cott, *The Bonds of Womanhood: "Woman's Sphere" in New England, 1780–1835* (New Haven, CT: Yale University Press, 1977).

82. Albert E. Mowry, *Sexual Instruction: Facts Versus Fancies* (Chicago: 1913), 5. Located in folder 5:10, Boys' Work, Kautz Family YMCA archives, University of Minnesota Libraries (hereafter Kautz Family YMCA Papers).

83. Bigelow, *Sex-Education*, 58.

84. Brumberg, *Body Project*, 16–17,

85. Bigelow, *Sex-Education*, 60–61.

86. See, for example, Faulkner and Carmichael, *Cottage Physician*, 546.

87. Margaret Cleaves, "Education in Sexual Hygiene for Young Working Women," *Charities and the Commons*, February 24, 1906, 8–12.

88. Ibid.

89. Both Kathy Peiss and Beth Bailey argue that working-class dating and heterosocial practices trickled up into the middle class in the Progressive Era. See Kathy Peiss, *Cheap Amusements: Working Women and Leisure in Turn-of-the-Century New York* (Philadelphia: Temple University Press, 1986); Beth Bailey, *From Front Porch to Back Seat: Courtship in Twentieth-Century America* (Baltimore: Johns Hopkins University Press, 1988). Paula Fass, in her examination of the 1920s, argues the reverse—that elite college students set the trends for acceptable sexual behavior. See Fass, *The Damned and the Beautiful: American Youth in the 1920s* (New York: Oxford University Press, 1977).

90. Lewis, *Gynecologic Consideration*. Lillian Faderman's work on the history of female romantic friendship sets Lewis's nonchalance in context; before a general acceptance of female sexuality in the early twentieth century, many authors and medical experts saw little of concern in female-female intimate relations. See Lillian Faderman, *Surpassing the Love of Men: Romantic Friendship and Love between Women from the Renaissance to the Present* (New York: William Morrow, 1981).

91. Lillian Faderman, *Odd Girls and Twilight Lovers: A History of Lesbian Life in Twentieth-Century America* (New York: Columbia University Press, 1991), 34; Leila J. Rupp, *A Desired Past: A Short History of Same-Sex Love in America* (Chicago: University of Chicago Press, 2002), 77.

92. Faderman, *Odd Girls and Twilight Lovers*; Smith-Rosenberg, *Disorderly Conduct*, chapter 2.

93. Bigelow, *Sex-Education*, 84–85.

94. Ibid., 154.

95. Canaday, *Straight State*, 30.

96. Hall, *Biology, Physiology and Sociology*, 129.

97. Hall, *Daughter, Mother and Father*, 5–9.

98. Daniel Walker Howe, "American Victorianism as a Culture," *American Quarterly* 27, no. 5 (1975): 530.

99. Alternate sources of "expertise" on childrearing, especially physicians and the press, were on the rise at this time period. See Apple, *Mothers and Medicine*.

100. Chesler, *Woman of Valor*, 69–70.

101. Margaret Sanger, *What Every Girl Should Know* (New York: M. N. Maisel, 1920).

102. Presumably, Sanger was referring to some schools that excused girls' absence from class once a month. Ibid., 26.

103. Margaret Sanger, *Family Limitation* (New York: 1914).

104. Margaret Sanger, "No Gods No Masters."

105. Clelia Duel Mosher, *Health and the Woman Movement* (New York: Young Women's Christian Association, 1916), 26.

106. Ibid., 44.

107. W. G. Tinckom Fernandez, "Y.W.C.A. Traveling Lecturer on Sex Hygiene," *Survey*, April 8, 1914, 76.

108. Nancy Marie Robertson, *Christian Sisterhood, Race Relations, and the YWCA, 1906–1946* (Champaign: University of Illinois Press, 2007), chapter 2.

109. *A Handbook for Leaders of Younger Girls*, Girls' Work Series (New York: Young Women's Christian Association, 1919), 10–11.

110. Ibid., 12.

111. Ibid., 27–29.

112. Susan A. Miller, "Girls in Nature / the Nature of Girls: Transforming Female Adolescence at Summer Camp, 1900–1939" (PhD diss., University of Pennsylvania, 2001), 29–30.

113. "Black History and the Girl Scouts of America," African American Registry, accessed November 25, 2014, http://www.aaregistry.org/historic_events/view/black-history-and-girl-scouts-america.

114. Girl Scouts of the USA, *Scouting for Girls: Official Handbook of the Girl Scouts*, 1st ed. (New York: Girl Scouts, 1920), 20.

115. W. J. Hoxie, *How Girls Can Help Their Country* (Bedford, MA: Applewood Books, 1913), vii, 28.

116. Helen Buckler, Mary Fielder, and Martha Allen, *Wo-He-Lo: The Story of the Camp Fire Girls 1910–1960* (New York: Holt, Rinehart & Winston, 1961).

117. Miller, "Girls in Nature," 38.

118. Charles A. Eastman, *Indian Scout Talks: A Guide for Boy Scouts and Camp Fire Girls* (Boston: Little, Brown, 1914), 148.

119. Several important studies show how the publication of VD rates of World War I recruits changed this almost instantly. See Bristow, *Making Men Moral*; Brandt, *No Magic Bullet*, chapter 2.

Chapter Four

1. Barnett M. Rhetta, "A Plea for the Lives of the Unborn," *Journal of the National Medical Association* 7, no. 3 (1915): 200–205.

2. "Md. Medic Gets Suspended Terms in Abortion Cases," *Jet Magazine*, July 7, 1955, 27.

3. "Jail 2 Baltimore Medics on Abortion Charges," *Jet Magazine* (14 April 1955), p. 25; "50-State Alert For Medic on Abortion Accusation," *Jet Magazine*, October 19, 1967, 23.

4. James Jones, *Bad Blood: The Tuskegee Syphilis Experiment* (New York: Free Press, 1981), chapter 2.

5. On the importance of race to progressivism in the South, see Woodward, *Origins of the New South*; Jack Temple Kirby, *Darkness at the Dawning: Race and Reform in the Progressive South* (Philadelphia: Lippincott, 1972); William A. Link, *The Paradox of Southern Progressivism, 1880–1930* (Chapel Hill: University of North Carolina Press, 1992); Gilmore, *Gender and Jim Crow*.

6. See, for example, Jessie M. Rodrique, "The Black Community and the Birth Control Movement," in *Passion and Power: Sexuality in History*, ed. Christina Simmons (Philadelphia: Temple University Press, 1989), 138–54; Christina Simmons, "African Americans and Sexual Victorianism in the Social Hygiene Movement, 1910–1940," *Journal of the History of Sexuality* 4, no. 1 (1993): 51–75; Johanna Schoen, *Choice and Coercion: Birth Control, Sterilization, and Abortion in Public Health and Welfare*. Chapel Hill: University of North Carolina Press, 2005.

7. It is important to recognize that "class" had both an economic meaning as well as one related to "respectability" and manners. See Mitchell, *Righteous Propagation*, chapters 3–4.

8. Sander Gilman's study of stereotypes of female anatomy and sexuality suggests that the exaggeration of African women's genitalia was used as a scientific tool to support the polygenetic belief that the races evolved from different beginnings. See Gilman, *Difference and Pathology*, chapter 3.

9. For the use of technology and scientific understanding, see Michael Adas, *Machines as the Measure of Men: Science, Technology, and Ideologies of Western Dominance* (Ithaca: Cornell University Press, 1989). Adas notes that by the height of African colonial expansion in the nineteenth century, race played a major role in Europeans' medical interpretation of Africans. Scientists made the same sorts of distinctions on issues of gender in the late nineteenth century. Scientists and medical men stressed women's smaller brain size and their reproductive systems as a justification for social policies that limited women's access to education and careers. Both the racial and gendered arguments of biological capacity dovetailed into the eugenics movement that gained popularity in the United States in the early twentieth century. For more on this, see Emily Martin, *The Woman in the Body: A Cultural Analysis of Reproduction* (Boston: Beacon Press, 1987); Laura Briggs, "The Race of Hysteria: 'Overcivilization' and the 'Savage' Woman in Late Nineteenth-Century Obstetrics and Gynecology," *American Quarterly* 52, no. 2 (2000): 246–73.

10. Hall, *Adolescence*.

11. Bederman, *Manliness and Civilization*, 28–29.

12. Megan Vaughan, *Curing Their Ills: Colonial Power and African Illness* (Stanford: Stanford University Press, 1991).

13. Laura Ann Stoler, *Race and the Education of Desire* (Durham, NC: Duke University Press, 1995); Eileen Findlay, *Imposing Decency: The Politics of Sexuality and Race in Puerto Rico, 1870–1920* (Durham, NC: Duke University Press, 1999). Whiteness studies also brings to mind the way racial and class identity were shaped in opposition to the "other." See particularly Roediger, *Wages of Whiteness*; Jacobson, *Whiteness of a Different Color*; Peter Kolchin, "Whiteness Studies: The New History of Race in America," *Journal of American History* 89, no. 1 (2002): 154–73.

14. Thomas Athol Joyce, "Negro," in *All There Is to Know: Readings from the Illustrious Eleventh Edition of the Encyclopedia Britannica*, ed. Charles Simmons (New York: Simon and Schuster, 1910), 245–46. Filipo Manetta was an Italian who published a volume in 1864 on the African race in America. See John S. Haller, *Outcasts from Evolution: Scientific Attitudes of Racial Inferiority, 1859–1900* (Urbana: University of Illinois Press, 1971), 36, 137.

15. Joyce, "Negro," 245–46.

16. See especially James G. Burrow, *AMA: Voice of American Medicine* (Baltimore: Johns Hopkins Press, 1963); James G. Burrow, *Organized Medicine in the Progressive Era* (Baltimore: Johns Hopkins University Press, 1977).

17. Howard W. Odum, *Social and Mental Traits of the Negro: Research into the Conditions of the Negro Race in Southern Towns* (New York: Columbia University Press, 1910), 38.

18. Ibid., 40.

19. The southern rape myth was white southerners' justification for lynching, arguing that black men constantly desired to rape white women. In fact, most of those who participated in lynchings never even claimed rape or attempted rape as a justification for their assaults on black men (and some black women). For more

on the southern rape myth, see Jacquelyn Dowd Hall, *Revolt against Chivalry: Jessie Daniel Ames and the Women's Campaign against Lynching* (New York: Columbia University Press, 1979); Patricia Ann Schechter, *Ida B. Wells-Barnett and American Reform, 1880–1930* (Chapel Hill: University of North Carolina Press, 2001).

20. Edward Bright Vedder, *Syphilis and Public Health* (Philadelphia: Lea & Febiger, 1918), 49.

21. Sander Gilman argues that scientists' emphasis of female genitalia reflects an assumption that while men of all races were not fundamentally different sexually, it was the allegedly vast difference between black and white women that illustrated the inequality the races. See Gilman, *Difference and Pathology*, 89–98.

22. Vedder, *Syphilis and Public Health*, 34.

23. Ibid., 32.

24. Charles Rosenberg and Janet Golden, eds., *Framing Disease: Studies in Cultural History* (New Brunswick, NJ: Rutgers University Press, 1992), xiii.

25. Kenneth M. Lynch, Kater McInnes, and G. Fleming McInnes, "Concerning Syphilis in the American Negro," *Southern Medical Journal* 8, no. 6 (1915): 450–56.

26. William Howard Lee, "The Negro as a Distinct Ethnic Factor in Civilization," *Medicine* 60 (1903): 424.

27. Henry McHatton, "The Sexual Status of the Negro—Past and Present," *American Journal of Dermatology and Genito-Urinary Diseases* 10, no. 1 (1906): 6.

28. Ibid. This question of slave health has been resurrected in the historiography, most notably in Robert William Fogel and Stanley Engerman, *Time on the Cross: The Economics of American Negro Slavery* (Boston: Little, Brown, 1974). For a refutation, see Herbert Gutman, *Slavery and the Numbers Game: A Critique of "Time on the Cross"* (Urbana: University of Illinois Press, 1975). For a more recent analysis of slavery and health, see Sharla M. Fett, *Working Cures: Healing, Health and Power on Southern Slave Plantations* (Chapel Hill: University of North Carolina Press, 2002).

29. McHatton, "Sexual Status," 8.

30. Ibid., 9.

31. Daniel David Quillian, "Racial Peculiarities: A Cause of the Prevalence of Syphilis in Negroes," *American Journal of Dermatology and Genito-Urinary Diseases* 10 (1906): 277.

32. Ibid.; McHatton, "Sexual Status," 9.

33. Quillian, "Racial Peculiarities," 277–78.

34. Elite southern whites had a paradoxical attitude toward black reproduction. Some hoped that African Americans would naturally "die out" through low birth rates, while others feared that a decrease in the African American population would threaten the South's labor supply.

35. McHatton, "Sexual Status," 9; Quillian, "Racial Peculiarities," 278. The data concerning the birth rate of African Americans is questionable, because of problems with the 1870 and 1880 census materials. Much has been made over the supposed drop in African American population after emancipation. In fact, the census data and subsequent studies demonstrate that there was not a drop in population, but rather a drop in the growth rate of the population. See also Linda Gordon, *Woman's Body, Woman's Right: A Social History of Birth Control in America* (New York: Grossman, 1976), 48, 151; Mitchell, *Righteous Propagation*, chapter 3.

36. Rodrique, "Black Community."

37. Mitchell, *Righteous Propagation*, 10–11; Susan L. Smith, *Sick and Tired of Being Sick and Tired: Black Women's Health Activism in America, 1890–1950* (Philadelphia: University of Pennsylvania Press, 1995).

38. Harriet A. Washington, *Medical Apartheid: The Dark History of Medical Experimentation on Black Americans from Colonial Times to the Present* (New York: Doubleday, 2006).

39. "An Interesting Book on the Negro," *Southern Medical Journal* 8, no. 4 (1915): 337.

40. "The Negro as a Factor in the Work of Preventive Medicine in the South," *Southern Medical Journal* 1, no. 6 (1908): 390.

41. "The National Health Week for Negroes," editorial, *Southern Medical Journal* 8, no. 8 (1915): 734.

42. Thomas W. Murrell, "Syphilis and the American Negro," *Journal of the American Medical Association* 54, no. 11 (1910): 847. Murrell was a lecturer on syphilis and dermatology at the University College of Medicine in Richmond, Virginia. Quillian also cites a similar finding but places the age of sexual experience for African American girls to be fourteen, rather than eighteen. See also Quillian, "Racial Peculiarities," 277.

43. Parker, *Articulating Rights*, 193; Deborah Gray White, *Too Heavy a Load: Black Women in Defense of Themselves, 1894–1994* (New York: W. W. Norton, 1999), 24.

44. John A. Kenney, "Syphilis and the American Negro—a Medico-Sociologic Study," *Journal of the National Medical Association* 1, no. 2 (1909): 115.

45. For a history of the National Medical Association, see Leonard E. Lawrence, "Why the NMA: Its Heritage Revisited and Future Challenges Assessed," *Journal of the National Medical Association* 85, no. 10 (1993): 745–48; Cynthia Charatz-Litt, "A Chronicle of Racism: The Effects of the White Medical Community on Black Health," *Journal of the National Medical Association* 84, no. 8 (1992): 717–25.

46. Frontispiece, *Journal of the National Medical Association* 1, no. 1 (January 1909).

47. John A. Kenney, "Salutatory," *Journal of the National Medical Association* 1, no. 2 (1909): 38.

48. Kenney, "Salutatory," 38.

49. White, *Too Heavy a Load*, 54.

50. For more on racial uplift, see Kevin K. Gaines, *Uplifting the Race: Black Leadership, Politics, and Culture in the Twentieth Century* (Chapel Hill: University of North Carolina Press, 1996); Gilmore, *Gender and Jim Crow*; Paula Giddings, *Where and When I Enter: The Impact of Black Women on Race and Sex in America* (New York: William Morrow, 1984), chapter 6; White, *Too Heavy a Load*.

51. Charles V. Roman, *American Civilization and the Negro: The Afro-American in Relation to National Progress* (Philadelphia: F. A. Davis, 1916), 47.

52. Gaines, *Uplifting the Race*.

53. C. V. Roman, "The Negro Woman and the Health Problem," *Journal of the National Medical Association* 7, no. 3 (1915): 185.

54. Roman was not alone in seeing interracial cooperation between women as the cornerstone of improved social and health policy. See Gilmore, *Gender and Jim Crow*, chapter 7; Smith, *Sick and Tired of Being Sick and Tired*; Evelyn Brooks Higginbotham, *Righteous Discontent: The Women's Movement in the Black Baptist Church, 1880–1920* (Cambridge, MA: Harvard University Press: 1993), chapter 4.

55. For an analysis of the black male critique of black women, see White, *Too Heavy a Load*, chapter 2.

56. Roman, "Negro Woman and the Health Problem," 189.

57. Ibid.

58. Ibid., 190.

59. Ibid., 189.

60. Ibid.

61. Historian Christina Simmons labels this "sexual Victorianism" and argues that it was an understandable response to the racial stereotypes of the period. See Simmons, "African Americans and Sexual Victorianism."

62. See Constance Chen, *The Sex Side of Life: Mary Ware Dennett's Pioneering Battle for Birth Control and Sex Education* (New York: New Press, 1996); Chesler, *Woman of Valor*; Gordon, *Woman's Body, Woman's Right*.

63. Sanger urged Americans to see contraception as a morally superior way to avoid abortion. See Chesler, *Woman of Valor*, 300–303.

64. Burwell, "Fertility of Women," 229.

65. Eleanor Alexander's analysis of the courtship of poets Paul Laurence Dunbar and Alice Ruth Moore notes how black prescriptive literature urged Moore and other elite black women to carefully select not just a life partner but the father of her children. See Eleanor Alexander, *Lyrics of Sunshine and Shadow: The Tragic Courtship and Marriage of Paul Laurence Dunbar and Alice Ruth Moore* (New York: New York University Press, 2001), 78–82.

66. Burwell, "Fertility of Woman," 228–29.

67. Mitchell, *Righteous Propagation*, 10–11.

68. L. L. Burwell, "The Fertility of Woman: Its Effects Physically and Morally upon the Nation," *Journal of the National Medical Association* 5, no. 4 (1913): 228.

69. Ibid., 229.

70. Rhetta, "Plea for the Lives of the Unborn," 202.

71. John A. Kenney, "Eugenics and the School Teacher," *Journal of the National Medical Association* 7, no. 4 (1915): 253–54.

72. Ibid., 257.

73. Giddings, *Where and When I Enter*, 137–38.

74. "Birth Control," *Journal of the National Medical Association* 9, no. 1 (1917): 98.

75. G. Jarvis Bowens, "Birth Control—as It Addresses Itself to the Physician," *Journal of the National Medical Association* 10, no. 4 (1918).

76. See, for example, "A Phase of Birth Control," *Journal of the National Medical Association* 12, no. 1 (1920): 31, C. V. Roman, "Some Ramifications of the Sexual Impulse," *Journal of the National Medical Association* 12, no. 1 (1920): 14–17.

77. For an overview of the American eugenics movement, see Mark Haller, *Eugenics: Hereditarian Attitudes in American Thought* (New Brunswick, NJ: Rutgers University Press, 1963); Donald Pickens, *Eugenics and the Progressives* (Nashville, TN: Vanderbilt Press, 1968); Daniel Kevles, *In the Name of Eugenics: Genetics and the Uses of Human Heredity* (New York: Knopf, 1985); Edward Larson, *Sex, Race, and Science: Eugenics in the Deep South* (Baltimore: Johns Hopkins University Press, 1995); Stern, *Eugenic Nation*.

78. For more on blacks and eugenics, see Jamie Hart, "Who Should Have the Children? Discussions of Birth Control among African-American Intellectuals, 1920–1939," *Journal of Negro History* 79, no. 1 (1994): 71–84.

79. It was later "discovered" by the mainstream press that the black community's skepticism about the aims of white physicians was rooted in fact. For two well-known examples, see Jones, *Bad Blood*; Rebecca Skloot, *The Immortal Life of Henrietta Lacks* (New York: Crown, 2010). For an overview of the roots of black distrust in the American health-care system, see Washington, *Medical Apartheid*.

80. Rhetta, "Plea for the Lives of the Unborn," 200.

81. Ibid., 203.

82. See also Dorothy E. Roberts, *Killing the Black Body: Race, Reproduction, and the Meaning of Liberty* (New York: Pantheon Books, 1997). For more on the complexity of women's agency and eugenic sterilization, see Schoen, *Choice and Coercion*.

83. Dr. Turner, "Vice Disease, Our Social and Economic Peril," *Journal of the National Medical Association* 5, no. 4 (1913): 250.

84. The construction of diseases as affecting only certain races or being a threat from certain races was prevalent in the Jim Crow South but also in immigration policy and concerns over Chinese immigration in San Francisco. See also Stern, *Eugenic Nation*, chapter 1; Nayan Shah, *Contagious Divides: Epidemics and Race in San Francisco's Chinatown* (Berkeley: University of California Press, 2001).

85. Peter F. Ghee, "Chronic Gonorrhoea," *Journal of the National Medical Association* 2, no. 2 (1910): 79.

86. Brandt, *No Magic Bullet*, 40.

87. "606," *Journal of the National Medical Association* 3, no. 1 (1911): 63.

88. "Lay Familiarity with 606," *Journal of the National Medical Association* 3, no. 2 (1911): 126.

89. Ghee, "Chronic Gonorrhoea," 77–78. While the brief articles do not mention specific dangers, it is true that Salvarsan 606, an arsenic compound, had dangerous side effects. An overdose can result in organ failure and death. Salvarsan was replaced by penicillin in the 1940s, which provided a safer and more effective treatment.

90. Darlene Clark Hine, "Rape and the Inner Lives of Black Women in the Middle West: Preliminary Thoughts on the Culture of Dissemblance," *Signs: Journal of Women in Culture and Society* 14, no. 4 (1988): 912–20.

91. The purity movement included several African American women like Frances E. W. Harper, who criticized the way slavery denied black women purity or male protection. See Parker, *Articulating Rights*, chapter 3; Parker, *Purifying America: Women, Cultural Reform, and Pro-censorship Activism, 1873–1933* (Urbana: University of Illinois Press, 1997), 47–48.

92. Stephanie Shaw, *What a Woman Ought to Be and to Do: Black Professional Women Workers during the Jim Crow Era* (Chicago: University of Chicago Press, 1996), 23.

93. Hine, "Rape and the Inner Lives of Black Women," 918.

94. For one such example, see Clayton E. Lust, "Confluence of Conflict: Houston and the Camp Logan Riot, 1917," unpublished essay in possession of the author.

95. Beverly Guy-Sheftall, "Sinner or Saint? Antithetical Views concerning Black Women and the Private Sphere," in *Daughters of Sorrow: Black Women in United States History* (Brooklyn: Carlson, 1990), 74–76.

96. White, *Too Heavy a Load*, chapter 2.

97. Higginbotham, *Righteous Discontent*, 193.

98. Willard B. Gatewood, *Aristocrats of Color: The Black Elite, 1880–1920* (Bloomington: Indiana University Press, 1990), chapter 7; Higginbotham, *Righteous Discontent.*

99. Quoted in Gatewood, *Aristocrats of Color,* 210. There is evidence, however, that Hope and Burns may not have practiced in private this public performance. For an alternate view, see Alexander, *Lyrics of Sunshine and Shadow,* chapter 4.

100. Alexander, *Lyrics of Sunshine and Shadow,* chapter 4.

101. Ibid., 99.

102. Sarah Delany, A. Elizabeth Delany, and Amy Hill Hearth, *Having Our Say: The Delany Sisters' First 100 Years* (New York: Dell, 1993), 57.

103. Ibid., 49.

104. Ruth Ann Stewart, *Portia: The Life of Portia Washington Pittman, the Daughter of Booker T. Washington* (Garden City, NY: Doubleday, 1977), 72.

105. Anastasia Curwood, *Stormy Weather: Middle-Class African American Marriages between the Two World Wars* (Chapel Hill: University of North Carolina Press, 2010), 3–7.

106. E. Azalia Hackley, *The Colored Girl Beautiful* (Kansas City, MO: Burton, 1916), 10–11. For more on advice literature for aspiring African Americans, see Mitchell, *Righteous Propagation,* chapter 4.

107. Ibid., 197. Alexander's survey of advice literature available to Paul Dunbar and Alice Moore also discusses the eugenic importance of good marriage and reproduction for race improvement. See Alexander, *Lyrics of Sunshine and Shadow,* 78–81.

108. Burwell, "Fertility of Woman," 228.

109. Ibid., 227–28.

110. Hackley, *Colored Girl Beautiful,* 45–46.

111. Ibid., 196.

112. Ibid., 112.

113. Hackley's manual was one of many sources of advice for young black women. For an analysis of black women's magazines from the late nineteenth and early twentieth centuries, see Noliwe M. Rooks, *Ladies' Pages: African American Women's Magazines and the Culture That Made Them* (New Brunswick, NJ: Rutgers University Press, 2004).

114. For more on black women's challenges to gender inequality, see Higginbotham, *Righteous Discontent,* chapter 5.

115. M. F. Armstrong, *On Habits and Manners* (Hampton: Normal School Press, 1888); R. C. O. Benjamin, *Don't: A Book for Girls* (San Francisco: Valleau & Peterson, Book and Job Printers, 1891).

116. Roman, *American Civilization and the Negro,* 69.

117. Joanna P. Moore, *"In Christ's Stead": Autobiographical Sketches* (Chicago: Women's Baptist Home Mission Society, 1902), 43.

118. Carter G. Woodson, *The Mis-education of the Negro* (Washington: Associated, 1933), especially 72.

119. Tera Hunter, *To 'Joy My Freedom: Southern Black Women's Lives and Labors after the Civil War* (Cambridge, MA: Harvard University Press, 1997), 143, 62; Higginbotham, *Righteous Discontent,* chapter 7.

120. See, for example, Hackley, *Colored Girl Beautiful,* 136; Gibson, Gibson, and Truitt, *Golden Thoughts*; Josie Briggs Hall, *Hall's Moral and Mental Capsule for*

the Economic and Domestic Life of the Negro, as a Solution of the Race Problem (Dallas: R. S. Jenkins, 1905), 5–13; Joseph R. Gay, *Life Lines of Success: A Practical Manual of Self Help for the Future Development of the Ambitious Colored American* (Chicago: W. R. Vansant, 1913), 318.

121. William Lee Howard, "The Negro as a Distinct Ethnic Factor in Civilization," *Medicine* 60 (1903): 423–26.

122. James Bardin, "Some Public Health Aspects of Race Relationships in the South," *Lectures and Addresses on the Negro in the South* (1915): 79–80.

123. Odum, *Social and Mental Traits*, 54.

124. Bederman, *Manliness and Civilization*, 28.

125. James McCulloch, ed., *Democracy in Earnest* (New York: Negro Universities Press, 1918), 321–25.

126. These ideas persisted well into the century, as anthropologists studying African American communities dismissed the moral influence churches may have held over their members. See, for example, John Dollard, *Caste and Class in a Southern Town* (New Haven, CT: Yale University Press, 1937), chapter 11. Hortense Powdermaker, *After Freedom: A Cultural Study in the Deep South* (New York: Viking Press, 1939), 162–64.

127. Moore, *"In Christ's Stead,"* 107. For a refutation of the supposed link between sexual immorality and slavery, see Gutman, *Black Family in Slavery and Freedom*.

128. E. Franklin Frazier, *The Negro Church in America* (New York: Schocken Books, 1963), 33–34. W. E. B. DuBois's study of black churches also notes both white and black criticism of sexual morality. See W. E. B. DuBois, "The Negro Church," in *DuBois on Religion*, ed. Phil Zuckerman (Walnut Creek: AltaMira Press, 1903), 135–37.

Chapter Five

1. War Department, *Annual Report of the Secretary of War for the Fiscal Year, 1918*, vol. 1 (Washington DC: Government Printing Office, 1918), 11. Only about two million served overseas.

2. George Walker, *Venereal Disease in the American Expeditionary Forces* (Baltimore: Medical Standard Book, 1922), 223.

3. On the connections between foreign ideologies and domestic reform, see Matthew Frye Jacobson, *Barbarian Virtues: The United States Encounters Foreign Peoples at Home and Abroad, 1876–1917* (New York: Hill and Wang, 2000).

4. William Johnson, "'Regulation' in the Philippines," *Woman's Journal*, November 10, 1900, 356.

5. For more on regulated prostitution in the United States, see Pivar, *Purity Crusade*, chapter 2.

6. Henry B. Blackwell, "Prostitution Licensed in the Philippines," *Woman's Journal*, September 1, 1900, 276.

7. For more on the history of prostitution and the American Army, see Holly A. Mayer, *Belonging to the Army: Camp Followers and Community during the American Revolution* (Columbia: University of South Carolina Press, 1996), 110–12. See also Bell Irvin Wiley, *The Life of Johnny Reb: The Common Soldier of the Confederacy* (Baton Rouge: Louisiana State University Press, 1943), 51–57; Bell Irvin Wiley, *The Life of*

Billy Yank: The Common Soldier of the Union (Baton Rouge: Louisiana State University Press, 1952), 257–62.

8. Aaron Belkin, *Bring Me Men: Military Masculinity and the Benign Façade of American Empire, 1898–2001* (New York: Columbia University Press, 2012), 128, 161.

9. L. M. Maus, "A Brief History of Venereal Diseases in the United States Army, and Measures Employed for their Suppression," June 14, 1917, folder 131:3, pp. 1–2, ASHA Papers.

10. For this argument, see also Pivar, *Purity and Hygiene*, 205.

11. Maus, "Brief History," 2.

12. Ibid., 5–6.

13. Ibid.

14. Ibid., 6.

15. Ibid., 7.

16. Frank E. Vandiver, *Black Jack: The Life and Times of John J. Pershing*, 2 vols. (College Station: Texas A&M Press, 1977), 2:662.

17. Pessimistic coverage of VD problems in the military was rampant in Progressive circles, although it did not reach a wide audience. For example, see Randall D. Warden, "Why Give Sex Instruction in High Schools," *Transactions of the Fourth International Congress on School Hygiene* 3 (1913): 180.

18. Raymond B. Fosdick, *Chronicle of a Generation: An Autobiography* (New York: Harper and Brothers, 1958), 138.

19. Ibid., 140.

20. *Report: YMCA Army and Navy Department*, July 13, 1916. Mexican Border Work, Kautz Family YMCA Papers.

21. *Report: Jerome D. Greene*, July 10, 1916. Mexican Border Work, Kautz Family YMCA Papers.

22. David Montejano, *Anglos and Mexicans in the Making of Texas* (Austin: University of Texas Press, 1987), 223–29; Molina, *Fit to Be Citizens*, chapters 2–3; Evelyn Nakano Glenn, *Unequal Freedom: How Race and Gender Shaped American Citizenship and Labor* (Cambridge, MA: Harvard University Press, 2002), 156; Neil Foley, "Partly Colored or Other White: Mexican Americans and Their Problems with the Color Line," in *Beyond Black and White: Race, Ethnicity, and Gender in the U.S. South and Southwest*, ed. Stephanie Cole and Alison M. Parker (College Station: Texas A&M University Press, 2004), 123–44.

23. Arnoldo de Leon, *They Called Them Greasers: Anglo Attitudes toward Mexicans in Texas, 1821–1900* (Austin: University of Texas Press, 1983), 36.

24. Ibid., 39–43.

25. Jacobson, *Whiteness of a Different Color*, 157–58.

26. Evelyn Nakano Glenn notes the dichotomy of stereotypes whites had about Mexican women, the oversexualized Mexican "spitfire" or the domestic drudge, and draws comparisons to the stereotypes of African American women as Jezebels or Mammies. Glenn, *Unequal Freedom*, 254–55.

27. W. H. Blodgett, "The Doctor on the Border—an Estimate of the Soldier Doctor and Incidents in the Life of the Border Soldier," *Indianapolis Medical Journal* 19 (1916): 431.

28. Blodgett's ideas were common among Californian health officials as well. See Molina, *Fit to Be Citizens*, chapter 2.

29. M. J. Exner, "Prostitution and Its Relation to the Army on the Mexican Border," *Journal of Social Hygiene* 3, no. 2 (1917): 218.

30. Ibid., 212.

31. Ibid., 205.

32. Ibid., 206.

33. Ibid., 209.

34. Ibid., 213.

35. Ibid., 214.

36. Ibid., 212.

37. Ibid., 218.

38. Exner's report did not reach a wide public audience, but was well known in military circles, according to Luther Gulick, another YMCA organizer active in the social hygiene movement. See Luther Gulick, *Morals and Morale* (New York: Association Press, 1919), 10.

39. Fosdick, *Chronicle of a Generation*, 141.

40. Quoted in Edward M. Coffman, *The War to End All Wars: The American Military Experience in World War I* (New York: Oxford University Press, 1968), 132–33. See also Fosdick, *Chronicle of a Generation*, 171; Hugh Young, *Hugh Young: A Surgeon's Autobiography* (New York: Harcourt, Brace, 1940), chapter 19.

41. Quoted in Fosdick, *Chronicle of a Generation*, 157.

42. Nancy K. Bristow's work includes numerous letters addressed to Wilson from citizens concerned about the moral health of the training camps. See Bristow, *Making Men Moral*, 1–3.

43. Newton Baker, *Frontiers of Freedom* (New York: George H. Doran, 1918), 94.

44. Woodrow Wilson also saw military action as a way to spread American hygiene across the globe. See Belkin, *Bring Me Men*, 132.

45. Bristow's monograph examining the Committee for Training Camp Activities makes this argument. She argues that neither the Progressive reformers nor the CTCA left a lasting legacy after the war. See Bristow, *Making Men Moral*.

46. Ibid., 8.

47. For a discussion of the American Plan in context of US policy toward prostitutes, see Pivar, *Purity and Hygiene*, chapter 9. Pivar argues that the social hygiene movement was split between the physician-dominated hygiene movement and the women-dominated purity movement; the war accelerated this factional split even while it institutionalized reform.

48. War Department Commission on Training Camp Activities, *Clean Communities Camps Fighters*, folder 131:4, ASHA Papers.

49. *News Bulletin #41*, National War Work Council, folder 4:14, Kautz Family YMCA Papers.

50. Charles Larned Robinson, *Don't Take a Chance*, Washington: War Department Commission on Training Camp Activities, folder 38:10, Armed Services Division Records, Kautz Family YMCA Archives.

51. Minutes, ASHA Annual Meeting, October 19, 1917, folder 5:6, ASHA Papers.

52. Raymond B. Fosdick, "Fit for Fighting—and After," *Scribner's*, April 1918, 415–23.

53. The term "white zone" is quoted in Gertrude Seymour, "The Health of Soldier and Civilian," *Survey*, April 24, 1918, 89.

54. Baker quoted in Ibid., 93.

55. Walker, *VD in the AEF*, 46–50.

56. Pivar, *Purity and Hygiene*.

57. Brandt, *No Magic Bullet*, 110–11.

58. Walker, *VD in the AEF*, 7. One should be cautious with Walker's statistics. VD statistics were still not uniformly taken, some including gonorrhea and some not, some only tallying active/infectious (rather than dormant) cases of syphilis.

59. Seymour, "Health of Soldier and Civilian," 93.

60. Quoted in Ronald H. Spector, "Josephus Daniels, Franklin Roosevelt, and the Reinvention of the Naval Enlisted Man," in *FDR and the U.S. Navy*, ed. Edward J. Marolda (New York: St. Martin's Press, 1998), 29.

61. Ronald Spector places Daniels's attitude toward prophylaxis within a larger goal of reforming the Navy into a respectable career. See ibid.

62. For more on the early purity movement, see Parker, *Purifying America*; Pivar, *Purity Crusade*; Walters, *Primers for Prudery*.

63. Jonathan Daniels, *The End of Innocence* (New York: Da Capo Press, 1972), chapter 2.

64. Walker, *VD in the AEF*, 219.

65. Fosdick, *Chronicle of a Generation*, 162.

66. Ibid., 162–63.

67. Gulick, *Morals and Morale*, 26.

68. United States Navy, *Live Straight If You Would Shoot Straight*, p. 15, folder 131:5, ASHA Papers.

69. Brandt, *No Magic Bullet*, 111. This is certainly an overestimate. See, for example, Edith Houghton Hooker, "A Criticism of Venereal Prophylaxis," *Journal of Social Hygiene* 4, no. 2 (1918).

70. *Notice to the Recruit and the Soldier in Regard to Venereal Diseases*, 1917, folder 170:6, ASHA Papers. Exner's study of prostitution during the Mexican Punitive Expedition gave soldiers six hours to receive treatment. See Exner, "Prostitution," 215.

71. *Shore Leave*, p. 2, folder 131:6, ASHA Papers.

72. Gulick, *Morals and Morale*, 27.

73. Quoted in Brandt, *No Magic Bullet*, 110.

74. Modern medical knowledge rejects this possibility, although the nineteenth- and early twentieth-century medical literature is replete with discussion of casual transmission of syphilis. See, for example, L. Duncan Bulkley, "Should Education in Sexual Matters Be Given to Young Men of the Working Classes?" *Charities and the Commons*, February 24, 1906, 5–8. For a historical analysis, see Laura Engelstein, "Morality and the Wooden Spoon: Russian Doctors View Syphilis, Social Class, and Sexual Behavior, 1890–1905," in *The Making of the Modern Body: Sexuality and Society in the Nineteenth Century*, ed. Thomas Walter Laqueur (Berkeley: University of California Press, 1987), 169–208.

75. Brandt, *No Magic Bullet*, 111.

76. Commission for Training Camp Activities, *Carry On*, n.d., folder 131:6, ASHA Papers. While there is no date provided, the story discusses a physician and soldier who had been at war for eighteen months, dating the piece to late 1918 or beyond.

77. Ibid., 6.

78. Ibid., 7.

79. Arthur E. Barbeau and Florette Henri, *The Unknown Soldiers, African-American Troops in World War I* (Philadelphia: Temple University Press, 1974), 36; Gerald E. Shenk, *Work or Fight! Race, Gender and the Draft in World War I* (New York: Palgrave, 2005).

80. Barbeau and Henri, *Unknown Soldiers*, 52–53.

81. Arthur B. Spingarn, "The War and Venereal Diseases among Negroes," *Journal of Social Hygiene* 4, no. 3 (1918): 336.

82. Ibid., 338. See also Barbeau and Henri, *Unknown Soldiers*, 54.

83. Spingarn, "War and Venereal Diseases among Negroes," 337. The problem of sterilization was not restricted to black troops. See Brandt, *No Magic Bullet*, 111. However, the attitude expressed by the surgeon demonstrates the deleterious effect racism could have on medical treatment.

84. Spingarn, "War and Venereal Diseases among Negroes," 338. For the lack of recreational facilities available to black troops, see also Barbeau and Henri, *Unknown Soldiers*, chapters 5–8; Mjagkij, *Light in the Darkness*, chapter 6.

85. Spingarn, "War and Venereal Diseases among Negroes," 341.

86. Mjagkij, *Light in the Darkness*, 86.

87. *Notes on the History of the Social Hygiene Division, Commission on Training Camp Activities, War and Navy Departments*, pp. 4–5, folder 131:3, ASHA Papers.

88. Ibid.

89. *Syllabus for Use in Lectures on Sex Hygiene and Venereal Disease*, 1918, pp. 4–5, folder 131:6, ASHA Papers.

90. Ibid., 3.

91. *Syllabus for Use in Lectures on Sex Hygiene and Venereal Diseases*, Washington, D.C., p. 11, folder 131:6, ASHA Papers.

92. YMCA National War Work Council, *News Bulletin #41*, October 1, 1917, p. 3, folder 4:14, Kautz Family YMCA Papers.

93. YMCA National War Work Council, *Social Hygiene Program*, n.d., pp. 3–4, folder 38:19, Kautz Family YMCA Papers.

94. Mjagkij, *Light in the Darkness*, 87–88.

95. *Notes on the History of the Social Hygiene Division*, pp., 6–7, folder 131:3, ASHA Papers.

96. William Aspenwall Bradley, "Work with Chaplains in the Army and Navy," *Journal of Social Hygiene* 4, no. 4 (1918): 443.

97. *Mail Bag* 3, ed. W. A. Bradley, August 31, 1918, p. 5, folder 131:7, ASHA Papers.

98. *Mail Bag* 4, September 28, 1918, p. 3.

99. *Mail Bag* 1, June 21, 1918, p. 2.

100. *Mail Bag* 4, September 28, 1918.

101. *Mail Bag* 1, June 21, 1918, p. 2.

102. Ibid., 3.

103. In civilian life as well, parents and physicians expressed concern that printed literature was more "seductive" than conversations. See Pierce, *What Adolescents Ought to Know*, 5–22.

104. The contradictory definitions of masculinity are at the heart of Aaron Belkin's work on military masculinity. See Belkin, *Bring Me Men*.

105. *Live Straight If You Would Shoot Straight*, p. 3, folder 131:5, ASHA Papers.

106. Ibid., 4.

107. *"Hello, Soldier Sport,"* folder 131:6, ASHA Papers.

108. *Shore Leave*, p. 2, folder 131:6, ASHA Papers.

109. *Notice to the Recruit and the Soldier in Regard to Venereal Diseases*, 1917, folder 170:6, ASHA Papers, 2.

110. *Home Reading Course for Citizen-Soldiers*, War Information Series 9 (Washington, DC: Committee on Public Information, 1917), 17.

111. Fred B. Smith, "Four Sins That Soldiers Say They Hate," *American Magazine*, November 1918, 131.

112. Ibid.

113. Elizabeth Shepley Sergent, "The Temper of the A. E. F.," *New Republic*, July 20, 1918, 337. The chaplain publication, the *Mail Bag*, also took issue with Smith's conclusions, using some of the same language. See *Mail Bag* 3, August 31, 1918, p. 1, folder 131:7, ASHA Papers.

114. For more on Progressives and efficiency, see Wiebe, *Search for Order*, chapter 6.

115. *"Hello, Soldier Sport,"* folder 131:6, ASHA Papers.

116. *Live Straight If You Would Shoot Straight*, folder 131:5, ASHA Papers, 5.

117. Robinson, *Don't Take a Chance*, Washington: War Department Commission on Training Camp Activities, folder 38:10, Armed Services Division Records, Kautz Family YMCA Archives.

118. *Live Straight If You Would Shoot Straight*, folder 131:5, ASHA Papers, 6.

119. See Rotundo, *American Manhood*, chapter 10; Filene, *Him/Her/Self*, chapters 3–4; Donald J. Mrozek, "From National Health to Personal Fulfillment, 1890–1940," in *Fitness in American Culture: Images of Health, Sport, and the Body, 1830–1940*, ed. Kathryn Grover (Amherst: University of Massachusetts Press, 1989), 18–46.

120. George Chauncey, *Gay New York: Gender, Urban Culture, and the Making of the Gay Male World, 1890–1940* (New York: Basic Books, 1994), 141–49.

121. While Canaday's quote was regarding soldiers during World War II, similar fears guided practice during World War I. Canaday, *Straight State*, chapter 2.

122. George Chauncey, "Christian Brotherhood or Sexual Perversion? Homosexual Identities and the Construction of Sexual Boundaries in the World War One Era," *Journal of Social History* 19 (1985): 189–211.

123. *Smash the Line!*, War Department Commission on Training Camp Activities, 1917, p. 16, folder 131:5, ASHA Papers.

124. Robinson, *Don't Take a Chance*, Washington: War Department Commission on Training Camp Activities, folder 38:10, Armed Services Division Records, Kautz Family YMCA Archives, 5.

125. *Live Straight If You Would Shoot Straight*, folder 131:5, ASHA Papers, 16.

126. William F. Snow and Wilbur A. Sawyer, "Venereal Disease Control in the Army," *Journal of the American Medical Association* 71, no. 6 (1918): 458.

127. Elizabeth Boies, "The Girls on the Border and What They Did for the Militia," *Social Hygiene* 3, no. 2 (1917): 221–28.

128. Mjagkij, *Light in the Darkness*, chapter 6.

129. The strategy and implementation of wholesome recreation will not be discussed at length here, as it is only tangentially related to sex education. For

an excellent analysis of this aspect of the American Plan, see Bristow, *Making Men Moral*. Bristow and others have noted that recreational facilities were also segregated, and that few if any programs were available to African American soldiers.

130. "Films for Sunday Night," "Educational Motion Pictures for the Camps," and "Build a Wall of Film about a Camp," folder 25:1, National War Work Council, Kautz Family YMCA Papers. For a list of films approved for military screenings, see Bristow, *Making Men Moral*, 225–26.

131. For more on patent medicine shows, see Ann Anderson, *Snake Oil, Hustlers and Hambones: The American Medicine Show* (Jefferson, NC: McFarland, 2000); James Harvey Young, *The Toadstool Millionaires: A Social History of Patent Medicines in America before Federal Regulation* (Princeton, NJ: Princeton University Press, 1961).

132. Anderson, *Snake Oil, Hustlers and Hambones*, 53. For more on anatomical museums, see Michael Sappol, "'Morbid Curiosity': The Decline and Fall of the Popular Anatomical Museum," *Common-Place* 4, no. 2 (2004), http://www.common-place.org/vol-04/no-02/sappol/.

133. Stereopticons were similar in concept to the Viewmaster toys of the twentieth century, in which two slides of different perspective are viewed together to create a three-dimensional visual effect.

134. "White Slavery on Film," *New York Times*, December 9, 1913, 8. Emphasis in original.

135. Ellis Paxon Oberholtzer, *The Morals of the Movies* (Philadelphia: Penn, 1922), 41–42.

136. H. C. Moore, "Report on the Committee on Study of Venereal Diseases," *Texas State Journal of Medicine* 12 (1917): 419.

137. H. E. K., "Sex Hygiene Exhibit for Recruits at Jefferson Barracks," *Texas State Journal of Medicine* 13 (1917): 191. A similar program was introduced in Fort Worth, Texas, using stereopticon slides furnished by the federal government. See also "Physician to Lecture to Soldiers Stationed at Fort Worth," *Texas State Journal of Medicine* 13 (1917): 193.

138. This description is based on numerous summaries of the film, including Brandt, *No Magic Bullet*, 68–70; Karl S. Lashley and John B. Watson, "A Psychological Study of Motion Pictures in Relation to Venereal Disease Campaigns," *Social Hygiene* 7, no. 2 (1921): 181–219. Dr. Martin Pernick of the University of Michigan assisted in locating the most complete information about these films.

139. Executive Committee minutes, 10 March 1919, folder 5:8, ASHA Papers.

140. Spector, "Josephus Daniels, Franklin Roosevelt, and the Reinvention of the Naval Enlisted Man," 29–30.

141. Quoted in *Mail Bag* 1, June 21, 1918, p. 4, folder 131:7, ASHA Papers.

142. Brandt, *No Magic Bullet*, 118–19. Debate persists among historians, as among moralists, as to whether the decrease was the result of moral or medical prophylaxis. Walker puts the rate by the Armistice at 35 per 1000. Walker, *VD in the AEF*, 101. Limiting access to prostitutes helped decrease VD rates, except for the Military Police who stood guard outside the French houses of prostitution. Military Police ironically had the highest rate of any category of soldiers. One French official stated, "Your police run the other boys away from the girls and then take them for themselves." Walker, *VD in the AEF*, 82–83.

Chapter Six

1. "Sauce for the Gander," *San Antonio Express*, March 3, 1918.

2. Exner, "Prostitution," 214.

3. I use Kathy Peiss's term, "charity girls," to represent a broad grouping of young women who, well before the war, began experimenting with sexual activity either in exchange for gifts and entertainment or for their own social and sexual fulfillment. See Peiss, *Cheap Amusements*, 110–13.

4. "Miss Miner Discusses Plans of the Committee on Protective Work for Girls, Created by the C. T. C. A.," *Social Hygiene Bulletin*, March 1918, folder 178:3, ASHA Papers.

5. Mabel S. Ulrich, *Mothers of America*, War Department, Commission on Training Camp Activities, folder 132: 7, ASHA Papers.

6. Ibid.

7. Ibid.

8. "What Is the Government Doing for Your Boy?" War Department, Commission on Training Camp Activities, n.d., folder 131:4, ASHA Papers.

9. Mrs. Woodallen Chapman, *The Nation's Call to Young Women*, War Department, Commission on Training Camp Activities, New York, 1918, folder 132:7, ASHA Papers.

10. Mrs. Woodallen Chapman, *Your Country Needs You*, War Department, Commission on Training Camp Activities, New York, folder 132:7, ASHA Papers.

11. Ibid.

12. *For a New World*, p. 9, folder 131:4, ASHA Papers.

13. See, for example, Theda Skocpol, *Protecting Soldiers and Mothers: The Political Origins of Social Policy in the United States* (Cambridge, MA: Belknap Press, 1992), part 3; Nancy Cott, *The Grounding of Modern Feminism* (New Haven, CT: Yale University Press, 1987).

14. *Why Our Women Are Frightened*, New York: Manger, Hughes and Manger, 1917. Located in Y-USA.4-1, folder 38:12, Kautz Family YMCA Papers.

15. Annette Kuhn, *Cinema, Censorship and Sexuality, 1909–1925* (London: Routledge, 1988), 52–53. Summary of the film plot comes from several sources, including "The End of the Road: The Story of a Motion Picture Drama Prepared for Women and Girls by the War Department," folder 131:8, ASHA Papers; American Film Institute, Catalog of Silent Films, accessed April 7, 2005, http://www.afi.com/members/catalog/silentHome.aspx?s=1.

16. Mary E. Odem, *Delinquent Daughters: Protecting and Policing Adolescent Female Sexuality in the United States, 1885–1920* (Chapel Hill: University of North Carolina Press, 1995), 22.

17. *The End of the Road*, folder 131:8, ASHA Papers.

18. John F. Piper, *The American Churches in World War I* (Athens: Ohio University Press, 1985), 137.

19. Lashley and Watson, "Psychological Study of Motion Pictures," 200.

20. Ibid., 181.

21. Ibid., 195.

22. Ibid., 204.

23. Ibid., 197.

24. Ibid., 211.

25. Oberholtzer, *Morals of the Movies*, 38.

26. Piper, *American Churches in World War I*, 157.

27. Oberholtzer, *Morals of the Movies*, 39.

28. Bristow, *Making Men Moral*, 190. For the return to the moralistic approach, see Lord, "Models of Masculinity."

29. The term "passionless" comes from Nancy Cott's work on nineteenth-century womanhood. See Cott, "Passionless."

30. Elizabeth Lunbeck, "'A New Generation of Women': Progressive Psychiatrists and the Hypersexual Female," *Feminist Studies* 13 (Autumn 1987): 514. On the medical discourse surrounding "abnormal" sexuality, see also Foucault, *History of Sexuality*.

31. For more on the construction of and reaction to "khaki fever," see Angela Woollacott, "'Khaki Fever' and Its Control: Gender, Class, Age and Sexual Morality on the British Homefront in the First World War," *Journal of Contemporary History* 29, no. 2 (1994): 325–47; Brandt, *No Magic Bullet*, 81–82; Miller, "Girls in Nature," 23–28.

32. Dock, *Hygiene and Morality*, 59.

33. Morrow, "Prophylaxis of Venereal Diseases," 663–69. For more on protection versus punishment of girls, see Judith Walkowitz, *Prostitution and Victorian Society: Women, Class, and the State* (Cambridge: Cambridge University Press, 1980), 249–56.

34. Hooker, "Criticism of Venereal Prophylaxis," 179.

35. Jennifer Lisa Koslow, *Cultivating Health: Los Angeles Women and Public Health Reform* (New Brunswick, NJ: Rutgers University Press, 2009), 134.

36. Kimberly Jensen, "Venereal Girls."

37. Hooker, "Criticism of Venereal Prophylaxis," 192.

38. Ibid., 191.

39. Harriet Hyman Alonso, *Peace as a Women's Issue: A History of the U.S. Movement for World Peace and Women's Rights* (Syracuse, NY: Syracuse University Press, 1993), chapter 3.

40. Aileen S. Kraditor, *The Ideas of the Woman Suffrage Movement, 1890–1920* (New York: Columbia University Press, 1965).

41. David Kennedy, *Over Here: The First World War and American Society* (New York: Oxford University Press, 1980), 284–87; Sara Evans, *Born for Liberty: A History of Women in America* (New York: Free Press, 1989), 170–72; Nancy Woloch, *Women and the American Experience* (New York: McGraw-Hill, 1994), 353; Kimberly Jensen, *Mobilizing Minerva: American Women in the First World War* (Urbana: University of Illinois Press, 2008).

42. Evans, *Born for Liberty*, 169–72.

43. Kathleen Kennedy, *Disloyal Mothers and Scurrilous Citizens: Women and Subversion during World War I* (Bloomington: Indiana University Press, 1999); Kim E. Nielsen, *Un-American Womanhood: Antiradicalism, Antifeminism, and the First Red Scare* (Columbus: Ohio State University Press, 2001), chapter 2.

44. Odem, *Delinquent Daughters*, 108; Koslow, *Cultivating Health*, 138. The federal government contributed well over $400,000 to detention homes and reformatories, including opening sixteen specifically for the wartime emergency and providing funding for twenty-seven existing homes. See Mary Macey Dietzler and Thomas A. Storey, *Detention Houses and Reformatories as Protective Social Agencies in the Campaign of*

the United States Government against Venereal Diseases (Washington, DC: Government Printing Office, 1922), 2.

45. Dietzler and Storey, *Detention Houses*, 11.

46. Brian Donovan, *White Slave Crusades: Race, Gender, and Anti-vice Activism, 1887–1917* (Urbana: University of Illinois Press, 2006), 138.

47. Dietzler and Storey, *Detention Houses*, 3; D'Emilio and Freedman, *Intimate Matters*, 212.

48. Brandt, *No Magic Bullet*, 90; Koslow, *Cultivating Health*, 145.

49. Odem, *Delinquent Daughters*, 1; Peiss, *Cheap Amusements*.

50. Mrs. Martha P. Falconer, "The Segregation of Delinquent Women and Girls as a War Problem," in *The Annals: War Relief Work*, ed. J. P. Lichtenberger (Philadelphia: American Academy of Political and Social Science, 1918), 166.

51. Dietzler and Storey, *Detention Houses*, 24–25. See also Kevin J. Mumford, *Interzones: Black/White Sex Districts in Chicago and New York in the Early Twentieth Century* (New York: Columbia University Press, 1997), chapter 6.

52. Ibid., 36.

53. Ibid., 68.

54. Cheryl Hicks, *Talk with You Like a Woman: African American Women, Justice, and Reform in New York, 1890–1935* (Chapel Hill: University of North Carolina Press, 2010), chapter 6. See also Faderman, *Odd Girls and Twilight Lovers*, 38.

55. Dietzler and Storey, Detention Houses, 214–15.

56. Ibid., 215.

57. Barbara Meil Hobson, *Uneasy Virtue: The Politics of Prostitution and the American Reform Tradition* (New York: Basic Books, 1987), 175.

58. Hugh Cabot, "Education Versus Punishment as a Remedy for Social Evils," *Fourth International Transactions of School Hygiene*, vol. 5, Buffalo, NY, August 25–30, 1913, 419.

59. Harrol B. Ayres, "Democracy at Work—San Antonio Being Reborn," *Journal of Social Hygiene* 4, no. 2 (1918): 211.

60. "The World Is Sizing Up San Antonio Which Has Jumped into Big League—London Told We Are 'the Wonder City,'" *San Antonio Express*, November 4, 1917.

61. "Law Enforcement Notes," *Social Hygiene Bulletin* 5, no. 4 (1918): 8.

62. Garna L. Christian, "Newton Baker's War on El Paso Vice," *Red River Valley Historical Review* 5, no. 2 (1980): 56. Christian details El Paso's failure to secure training camps because of the town's poor record fighting prostitution. See also Ann R. Gabbert, "Prostitution and Moral Reform in the Borderlands: El Paso, 1890–1920," *Journal of the History of Sexuality* 12, no. 4 (2003): 575–604.

63. "San Antonio Realty Now on Safe and Solid Basis," *San Antonio Express*, October 14, 1917.

64. "New Year Sees Prosperity and Population of 250,000," *San Antonio Express*, January 1, 1918.

65. "The War and San Antonio," *San Antonio Express*, January 27, 1918.

66. "Morale Depends on Morality, Says Rev. S. J. Porter," *San Antonio Express*, January 7, 1918.

67. "Commanders Urge City to Clean Up," *San Antonio Express*, January 5, 1918.

68. "Camp Commanders Urge San Antonio to Clean Up and Avert Action," *San Antonio Express*, January 5, 1918.

69. This is true for reformers across the country. See Peggy Pascoe, *Relations of Rescue: The Search for Female Moral Authority in the American West, 1874–1939* (New York: Oxford University Press, 1990).

70. "Appointment of Policewomen Is Urged by Women," *San Antonio Express*, December 14, 1917.

71. "Biographical Summary of Mrs. LeRoy Sumner Bates," folder 1:8, Woman's Club of San Antonio Records, 1898–1994, MS 1, UTSA Archives, Library, University of Texas at San Antonio (hereafter cited as WCSA Records).

72. "The Women Have Spoken," *San Antonio Express*, December 1, 1917. For more on patriotic motherhood, see also Kennedy, *Disloyal Mothers*.

73. "War Department to Protect Girls," *San Antonio Express*, November 6, 1917.

74. Outcry over corrupt male politicians and police officers was ubiquitous in the editorials and media coverage of the vice crusade. For example, there was intense newspaper coverage of the trial of Chief of Police Fred H. Lancaster and judge of the Corporation Court, J. Ed Wilkens, who were charged with excessive leniency in vice cases. Both were cleared of charges, which only increased media reaction. See, for example, "Chief and Judge Found Not Guilty by City Council," *San Antonio Express*, January 12, 1918; "Captain and Two Officers in Vice Squad Suspended," *San Antonio Express*, March 7, 1918; "Vice Squad Head and Detectives Are Discharged," *San Antonio Express*, April 10, 1918.

75. "Women of City in Vice Crusade Ask for Policewomen," *San Antonio Express*, December 1, 1917.

76. Bettye Womack, "Introduction," folder 1:6, WCSA Records.

77. Gloria Myers, *A Municipal Mother: Portland's Lola Greene Baldwin, America's First Policewoman* (Corvallis: Oregon State University Press, 1995).

78. "Minute Books, 1910–1914," folder 24:1, WCSA Records; "Board of Directors' Notes," folder 9:36, WCSA Records.

79. "Women of City in Vice Crusade Ask for Policewomen," *San Antonio Express*, December 1, 1917.

80. "Appointment of Policewomen Is Urged by Women"; "Women on Police Force," *San Antonio Express*, December 26, 1917; Myers, *Municipal Mother*.

81. "Women Police," *San Antonio Express*, December 15, 1917.

82. "Six Local Women Given Power of City Policemen," *San Antonio Express*, December 28, 1917.

83. "Fifteen Deputy Policewomen Are Asked of Mayor," *San Antonio Express*, January 7, 1918.

84. "Police Watching Rooming Houses," *San Antonio Express*, January 15, 1918.

85. "Six Local Women Given Power of City Policemen," *San Antonio Express*, December 28, 1917.

86. "'No Man's Land' Unsafe for Women or Men in City," *San Antonio Express*, January 9, 1918.

87. "Policewomen Are Out; Law Creating Offices Repealed," *San Antonio Express*, February 1, 1918.

88. Rena M. Green, "The Dismissal of the Women Police," *San Antonio Express*, February 2, 1918.

89. "Strongly Protest Summary Release of 6 Policewomen," *San Antonio Express*, February 6, 1918.

NOTES TO PP. 124–127

90. Francesco Cordasco and Thomas Monroe Pitkin, *The White Slave Trade and the Immigrants: A Chapter in American Social History* (Detroit: Blaine Ethridge, 1981), 4–5.

91. Judge's Docket Book 9, 1917–18, Bexar County Courthouse, San Antonio, Texas. It is sometimes difficult to determine which charges were related to prostitution, as many unspecific charges could be applied for those purposes. For my research, I include charges such as "Keeping a disorderly house" and "Being a common prostitute," but not unspecific charges like "Vagrancy."

92. "Vice Squad's 34 Arrests Bring $855 Fines to City," *San Antonio Express*, January 10, 1918; "Vice Squad Lands Fourteen in Cells," *San Antonio Express*, February 13, 1918.

93. "Fines Assessed Pay Salaries of City Vice Squad," *San Antonio Express*, May 6, 1918.

94. "Mujeres Detenidas Por Rijosas," *La Prensa*, November 7, 1917.

95. "Treinta Y Cinco Negros Aprehendidos Por Vagos," *La Prensa*, November 24, 1917.

96. José E. Limón, "Tex-Sex-Mex: American Identities, Lone Stars, and the Politics of Racialized Sexuality," *American Literary History* 9, no. 3 (1997): 598–616.

97. Neil Foley, *The White Scourge: Mexicans, Blacks, and Poor Whites in Texas Cotton Culture* (Berkeley: University of California Press, 1997). For distinctions in racial identity and the strategic adoption of white identity, see also Guadalupe San Miguel, *Let All of Them Take Heed: Mexican Americans and the Campaign for Educational Equality in Texas, 1910–1981* (Austin: University of Texas Press, 1987).

98. "Fifteen Arrests Made by Police," *San Antonio Express*, April 4, 1918; Judge's Docket Books 9–10, 1917–18, Bexar County Courthouse, San Antonio, Texas.

99. See, for example, "Mujeres Rijosas," *La Prensa*, April 20, 1918; "Once Aprehensiones," *La Prensa*, April 27, 1918. The term "ill women" may have signified carriers of venereal diseases.

100. Case 13314: *The State of Texas vs. Mrs. Annie Lacey*, October 10, 1917, Bexar County Courthouse, San Antonio, Texas.

101. "War Department Given Pledge City Will Be Cleaned," *San Antonio Express*, November 22, 1917. Reformers used the term "menace" to describe both VD and VD-infected women. See also Falconer, "Segregation of Delinquent Women and Girls as a War Problem," 160, 66; Katherine Bement Davis, "Women's Education in Social Hygiene," in *The Annals: War Relief Work*, ed. J. P. Lichtenberger (Philadelphia: American Academy of Political and Social Science, 1918), 169.

102. "Many Arrests by Army Police for Law's Violation," *San Antonio Express*, March 14, 1918.

103. Vagrancy charges against black women spoke not just to sexual impropriety but also to a postemancipation effort by whites to define black women as laborers. See Linda K. Kerber, *No Constitutional Right to Be Ladies: Women and the Obligations of Citizenship* (New York: Hill and Wang, 1998), chapter 2.

104. "64 Negro Women Arrested in Raid," *San Antonio Express*, March 14, 1918.

105. Dietzler and Storey, *Detention Houses*, 174–77.

106. Advertisement, *San Antonio Express*, December 4, 1917.

107. "Biographical Summary of Mrs. LeRoy Sumner Bates," folder 1:8, WCSA Records; "Yearbooks, 1917–1918," folder 2:2, WCSA Records.

108. D'Emilio and Freedman, *Intimate Matters*, 212.

109. See, for example, Linda Gordon, *Pitied but Not Entitled: Single Mothers and the History of Welfare, 1890–1935* (New York: Free Press, 1994); Kraditor, *Woman Suffrage Movement*.

110. For other case studies on detention homes, see Koslow, *Cultivating Health*, chapter 5; Jensen, "Venereal Girls." Jensen notes that while the Cedars case files specify Negro women, she has yet to uncover any evidence of Chinese American detainees. More research needs to be done to analyze racial politics in the Pacific Northwest.

111. De Leon, *They Called Them Greasers*, 39–44; D'Emilio and Freedman, *Intimate Matters*, 107–8; Stoler, *Race and the Education of Desire*, 8–11.

Chapter Seven

1. Walker, *VD in the AEF*, 2.

2. *Carrying on in Times of Peace*, War Department Commission on Training Camp Activities, folder 131:4, ASHA Papers.

3. Walker, *VD in the AEF*, 43.

4. Ibid.

5. Wilbur A. Sawyer, "Venereal Disease Control in the Military Forces," *American Journal of Public Health* 9, no. 5 (1919): 345.

6. Raymond Fosdick, "Fit for Fighting—and After," *Scribner's*, April 1918, 415–23.

7. "War on Venereal Disease to Continue," folder 131:4, ASHA Papers.

8. Ulysses Lee, *The Employment of Negro Troops* (Washington, DC: Government Printing Office, 2000), 3–5.

9. Addie W. Hunton and Kathryn M. Johnson, *Two Colored Women with the American Expeditionary Forces* (Brooklyn: Brooklyn Eagle Press, 1920), 186.

10. Ibid., 188.

11. Ibid., 173.

12. Ibid., 189.

13. For more on American assumptions about "French" identity and sexuality, see Alecia P. Long, *The Great Southern Babylon: Sex, Race, and Respectability in New Orleans, 1865–1920* (Baton Rouge: Louisiana State University Press, 2004). Long notes that in American commercial sex parlance, "French" referred to a woman's willingness to perform oral sex rather than her ethnic origin.

14. Falconer, "Segregation of Delinquent Women and Girls as a War Problem," 160.

15. Bristow, *Making Men Moral*, 192–98.

16. Jane Deeter Rippin, "Social Hygiene and the War," *Journal of Social Hygiene* 5 (1919): 125–36.

17. Jensen, "Venereal Girls."

18. Koslow, *Cultivating Health*, 151–54.

19. "News," *Texas State Journal of Medicine* 15 (August 1919): 163; Dietzler and Storey, *Detention Houses*, 175.

20. Lord, "Naturally Clean and Wholesome," 426–28; Moran, *Teaching Sex*, 74.

21. "Amended Budget 1919–1920," folder 5:8; "Budget for 1921–1922," folder 6:1; "First Draft of Budget for 1922–1923," folder 6:2; "Analysis of Budget for 1923–24," folder 6:3, ASHA Papers.

22. Gertrude Hefferan to Raymond Fosdick, January 8, 1921, folder 25:9, ASHA Papers.

23. Warren G. Harding, "Back to Normal: Address Before Home Market Club," Boston, Massachusetts, May 14, 1920.

24. For more on political dissent during the 1920s, see Nielsen, *Un-American Womanhood*.

25. Mumford, *Interzones*, part 2.

26. For a nuanced analysis of interracial sexual and romantic relationships in the South, see Charles F. Robinson II, *Dangerous Liaisons: Sex and Love in the Segregated South* (Fayetteville: University of Arkansas Press, 2003).

27. Mumford, *Interzones*.

28. United States Public Health Service, *Keeping Fit*, 1919, posters 29 and 30. ASHA Papers.

29. Lord, *Condom Nation*, 39.

30. United States Public Health Service, *Youth and Life*, 1920, posters 17 and 26. ASHA Papers.

31. United States Public Health Service, *Annual Report of the Surgeon General of the Public Health Service of the United States* (Washington, DC: Government Printing Office, 1921), 376–77.

32. For an extensive examination of the Public Health Service's efforts, see Lord, *Condom Nation*, especially 37–42.

33. For more on the failures of female passionlessness, see Lord, "Naturally Clean and Wholesome"; Frances Isabel Davenport, *Salvaging of American Girlhood: A Substitution of Normal Psychology for Superstition and Mysticism in the Education of Girls* (New York: E. P. Dutton, 1924).

34. William J. Fielding, *What Every Young Woman Should Know* (Girard, Kansas: Haldeman-Julius, 1924). Pierce, *What Adolescents Ought to Know*, 149–50.

35. The "sexual revolution" was more in media coverage than in behaviors and attitudes. Young people in the 1920s believed they were acting in a revolutionary manner, even if their behavior was not so distinct from the previous generation's. See Paula Fass, *Damned and the Beautiful*, chapter 6.

36. Jones, *Alfred C. Kinsey*, 321–23. Moran, *Teaching Sex*, 89–97; Freeman, *Sex Goes to School*, chapter 2. Freeman notes that by midcentury, the marital life model dominated American sex education.

37. Moran, *Teaching Sex*, 93.

38. Freeman, *Sex Goes to School*, 6; Moran, *Teaching Sex*, 105. Moran notes that these numbers are undoubtedly high, as schools that failed to respond to the survey on sex education were probably less likely to offer sex education.

39. Moran, *Teaching Sex*, 108–9.

40. Martha H. Verbrugge, *Active Bodies: A History of Women's Physical Education in Twentieth-Century America* (New York: Oxford University Press, 2012).

41. Brumberg, *Body Project*, 46.

42. Pierce, *What Adolescents Ought to Know*, 149.

43. Margaret Sanger, *Woman and the New Race* (New York: Truth, 1920), 151.

44. Chesler, *Woman of Valor*, 484.

45. Faderman, *Odd Girls and Twilight Lovers*, 54.

46. Martha H. Verbrugge, *Active Bodies: A History of Women's Physical Education in Twentieth-Century America* (New York: Oxford University Press, 2012).

47. Joshua Zeitz, *Flapper: A Madcap Story of Sex, Style, Celebrity, and the Women Who Made America Modern* (New York: Three Rivers Press, 2006).

48. Frank Walsh, *Sin and Censorship: The Catholic Church and the Motion Picture Industry* (New Haven, CT: Yale University Press, 1996), 12–13; Gregory D. Black, *Hollywood Censored: Morality Codes, Catholics, and the Movies* (Cambridge: Cambridge University Press, 1994), 37; Parker, *Purifying America*, chapter 5.

49. Walsh, *Sin and Censorship*, chapters 1–2; Black, *Hollywood Censored*, chapter 1.

50. Black, *Hollywood Censored*, 305. The Lord-Quigley proposal became the basis for the Hays Code in 1930.

51. Walsh, *Sin and Censorship*, 20–21.

52. For more, see David Levering Lewis, *When Harlem Was in Vogue* (New York: Oxford University Press, 1979), 162–65. Heterosexuals also delved into exotic fantasy when "slumming" in homosexual bars in New York during the early twentieth century. See Chauncey, *Gay New York*, 36–41.

53. Chapman, *Prove It on Me*, chapter 3.

54. Ad Access On-Line Project—Ad #BH0281, John W. Hartman Center for Sales, Advertising & Marketing History, David M. Rubenstein Rare Book & Manuscript Library, http://library.duke.edu/digitalcollections/adaccess.

55. Brumberg, *Body Project*, 46.

56. Ad Access On-Line Project—Ad #BH0024, John W. Hartman Center for Sales, Advertising & Marketing History, David M. Rubenstein Rare Book & Manuscript Library, http://library.duke.edu/digitalcollections/adaccess.

57. Ad Access On-Line Project—Ad #BH0018, John W. Hartman Center for Sales, Advertising & Marketing History, David M. Rubenstein Rare Book & Manuscript Library, http://library.duke.edu/digitalcollections/adaccess.

58. Edward Behr, *Prohibition: Thirteen Years That Changed America* (New York: Arcade, 1996), 47–50.

Conclusion

1. See, for example, Burnham, "Progressive Era Revolution"; Ullman, *Sex Seen*; Kevin White, *The First Sexual Revolution: The Emergence of Male Heterosexuality in Modern America* (New York: New York University Press, 1993).

2. Belkin, *Bring Me Men*, 178–79.

3. Dana Ford, "Chambliss' Comments on Sexual Assault," *CNN.com*, June 5, 2013, http://www.cnn.com/2013/06/04/politics/chambliss-sexual-assaults.

4. Carter, *Heart of Whiteness*.

5. Jane Dailey, "The Theology of Massive Resistance: Sex, Segregation, and the Sacred after *Brown*," in *Massive Resistance: Southern Opposition to the Second Reconstruction*, ed. Clive Webb (Oxford: Oxford University Press, 2005): 151–80.

6. Pablo Mitchell, *West of Sex: Making Mexican America, 1900–1930* (Chicago: University of Chicago Press, 2012), introduction.

7. Danielle McGuire, *At the Dark End of the Street: Black Women, Rape, and Resistance—a New History of the Civil Rights Movement from Rosa Parks to the Rise of Black Power* (New York: Knopf, 2010).

8. Boston Women's Health Book Collective, *Our Bodies, Ourselves* (New York: Simon & Schuster, 1973).

9. Lisa McGirr, *Suburban Warriors: The Origins of the New American Right* (Princeton, NJ: Princeton University Press, 2001), 227–31.

10. Moran, *Teaching Sex*, chapter 6; Janice Irvine, *Talk about Sex: The Battle over Sex Education in the United States* (Berkeley, University of California Press, 2004).

11. Robinson, *Sex Knowledge for Men*, 4.

12. Julian B. Carter, "Birds, Bees, and Venereal Disease: Toward an Intellectual History of Sex Education," *Journal of the History of Sexuality* 10, no. 2 (2001): 213–49; United States House of Representatives Committee on Government Reform—Minority Staff, *The Content of Federally Funded Abstinence-Only Education Programs* (report prepared for Rep. Henry A. Waxman), 2004.

13. See, for example, Pamela K. Kohler, Lisa E. Manhart, William T. Lafferty, "Abstinence-Only and Comprehensive Sex Education and the Initiation of Sexual Activity and Teen Pregnancy," *Journal of Adolescent Health* 42, no. 4 (April 2008), 344–51.

14. Allan Brandt argues that the first generation of health reformers like Fournier expressed the goal of teaching women about sexuality not for their own benefit or health but for that of their children. See Brandt, *No Magic Bullet*, 16.

15. Lord, *Condom Nation*, chapter 7.

16. Sarah Kliff, "Rep. Todd Akin Is Wrong about Rape and Pregnancy, but He's Not Alone," *Washington Post Online*, August 20, 2012, http://www.washingtonpost.com/blogs/wonkblog/wp/2012/08/20/rep-todd-akin-is-wrong-about-rape-and-pregnancy-but-hes-not-alone/.

17. G. Stanley Hall, "Sex Hygiene in Infantile and Pre-pubertal Life," in *Transactions of the Fourth International Congress on School Hygiene* (Buffalo, NY, 1913), 4:14. For more on G. Stanley Hall's biological and cultural understandings of gender, see Bederman, *Manliness and Civilization*, chapter 3.

18. Willson, "Outline Program," 3:36.

Bibliography

Manuscript Collections

Ad*Access On-Line Project. John W. Hartman Center for Sales, Advertising & Marketing History. Duke University. David M. Rubenstein Rare Book & Manuscript Library. http://library.duke.edu/digitalcollections/adaccess.

American Social Hygiene Association Papers. Social Welfare History Archives Center. University of Minnesota, Minneapolis, Minnesota.

Bexar County Courthouse Records, San Antonio, Texas.

Kautz Family YMCA Archives. University of Minnesota Libraries, Minneapolis, Minnesota.

Woman's Club of San Antonio Records. UTSA Archives. Library, University of Texas at San Antonio.

Primary Sources

Addams, Jane. *Twenty Years at Hull-House*. New York: Macmillan, 1910.

Antin, Mary. *The Promised Land*. Boston: Houghton Mifflin, 1912.

Armstrong, M. F. *On Habits and Manners*. Hampton: Normal School Press, 1888.

Ayres, Harrol B. "Democracy at Work—San Antonio Being Reborn." *Journal of Social Hygiene* 4, no. 2 (1918): 211–17.

Baker, Newton. *Frontiers of Freedom*. New York: George H. Doran, 1918.

Bardin, James. "Some Public Health Aspects of Race Relationships in the South." *Lectures and Addresses on the Negro in the South* (1915): 70–83.

Benjamin, R. C. O. *Don't: A Book for Girls*. San Francisco: Valleau & Peterson, Book and Job Printers, 1891.

Bigelow, Maurice A. *Sex-Education: A Series of Lectures Concerning the Knowledge of Sex in Its Relation to Human Life*. New York: Macmillan, 1916.

"Birth Control." *Journal of the National Medical Association* 9, no. 1 (1917): 93–94.

Blackwell, Elizabeth. *The Laws of Life with Special Reference to the Physical Education of Girls*. New York: G. P. Putnam, 1852.

Blackwell, Henry B. "Prostitution Licensed in the Philippines." *Woman's Journal*, September 1, 1900.

Bliven, Bruce. "Flapper Jane." *New Republic*, September 9, 1925, 65–67.

Blodgett, W. H. "The Doctor on the Border—an Estimate of the Soldier Doctor and Incidents in the Life of the Border Soldier." *Indianapolis Medical Journal* 19 (1916): 429–33.

Boies, Elizabeth. "The Girls on the Border and What They Did for the Militia." *Social Hygiene* 3, no. 2 (1917): 221–28.

Boston Women's Health Book Collective. *Our Bodies, Ourselves.* New York: Simon & Schuster, 1973.

Bowens, G. Jarvis. "Birth Control—as It Addresses Itself to the Physician." *Journal of the National Medical Association* 10, no. 4 (1918): 176–78, appendix p. xix.

Boy Scouts of America (BSA). *Handbook for Scout Masters, Boy Scouts of America.* New York: BSA, 1914.

———. *The Official Handbook for Boys.* New York: Doubleday, 1913.

Bradley, William Aspenwall. "Work with Chaplains in the Army and Navy." *Journal of Social Hygiene* 4, no. 4 (1918): 443–52.

Bulkley, L. Duncan. "Should Education in Sexual Matters Be Given to Young Men of the Working Classes?" *Charities and the Commons*, February 24, 1906, 5–8.

Burwell, L. L. "The Fertility of Woman: Its Effects Physically and Morally upon the Nation." *Journal of the National Medical Association* 5, no. 4 (1913): 228.

Cabot, Hugh. "Education Versus Punishment as a Remedy for Social Evils." *Fourth International Transactions of School Hygiene*, vol. 5. Buffalo, NY. August 25–30, 1913, 35–44.

Clarke, Edward. *Sex in Education, or a Fair Chance for Girls.* Boston: Harvard University Press, 1873.

Cleaves, Margaret. "Education in Sexual Hygiene for Young Working Women." *Charities and the Commons*, February 24, 1906, 8–12.

Davenport, Frances Isabel. *Salvaging of American Girlhood: A Substitution of Normal Psychology for Superstition and Mysticism in the Education of Girls.* New York: E. P. Dutton, 1924.

Davis, Katharine Bement. *Factors in the Sex Life of Twenty-Two Hundred Women.* New York: Harper & Brothers, 1929.

———. "Women's Education in Social Hygiene." In *The Annals: War Relief Work*, edited by J. P. Lichtenberger, 167–77. Philadelphia: American Academy of Political and Social Science, 1918.

De Costa, B. E. "The White Cross Movement." *Philanthropist* 1, no. 1 (1886): 1–2.

Dietzler, Mary Macey, and Thomas A. Storey. *Detention Houses and Reformatories as Protective Social Agencies in the Campaign of the United States Government against Venereal Diseases.* Washington, DC: Government Printing Office, 1922.

Dock, Lavinia. *Hygiene and Morality: A Manual for Nurses and Others, Giving an Outline of the Medical, Social, and Legal Aspects of Venereal Diseases.* New York: G. P. Putnam's Sons, 1910.

Dollard, John. *Caste and Class in a Southern Town.* New Haven, CT: Yale University Press, 1937.

Douglass, H. Paul. *How Shall the Country Youth Be Served? A Study of "Rural" Work of Certain Character-Building Agencies.* New York: George H. Doran, 1926.

DuBois, W. E. B. "The Negro Church." In *DuBois on Religion*, edited by Phil Zuckerman, 45–46. Walnut Creek: AltaMira Press, 1903.

Eastman, Charles A. *Indian Scout Talks: A Guide for Boy Scouts and Camp Fire Girls.* Boston: Little, Brown, 1914.

Eliot, Charles W. "The American Social Hygiene Association." *Social Hygiene* 1, no. 1 (1914): 1–5.

———. *The Training for an Effective Life.* Boston: Houghton Mifflin, 1915.

Eliot, Thomas D. "Social Hygiene at the Panama-Pacific International Exposition." *Journal of Social Hygiene* 1, no. 3 (1915): 397–414.

Exner, M. J. "Prostitution and Its Relation to the Army on the Mexican Border." *Journal of Social Hygiene* 3, no. 2 (1917): 205–20.

———. "Sex Education Literature for Boys and Men." *American Youth* 2, no. 1 (1913): 74–84.

Falconer, Mrs. Martha P. "The Segregation of Delinquent Women and Girls as a War Problem." In *The Annals: War Relief Work*, edited by J. P. Lichtenberger, 160–66. Philadelphia: American Academy of Political and Social Science, 1918.

Faulkner, Thomas, and J. H. Carmichael. *The Cottage Physician: Best Known Methods of Treatment in All Diseases, Accidents and Emergencies of the Home.* Springfield, MA: King, Richardson, 1892.

Fernandez, W. G. Tinckom. "Y.W.C.A. Traveling Lecturer on Sex Hygiene." *Survey*, April 8, 1914, 76.

Fielding, William J. *What Every Young Woman Should Know.* Girard, Kansas: Halde-man-Julius Company, 1924.

Filler, Louis. *Muckraking and Progressivism in the American Tradition.* New Brunswick, NJ: Transaction Press, 1996.

Finn, A. H. "Detroit Sex Hygiene Campaign." *Survey*, December 17, 1910, 460–61.

Fisher, George J. "Sex Education in the Young Men's Christian Association." *Journal of Social Hygiene* 1, no. 2 (1915): 226–30.

Forbush, William Byron. *The Boy Problem: A Study in Social Pedagogy.* Boston: Pilgrim Press, 1901.

Ford, Dana. "Chambliss' Comments on Sexual Assault." *CNN.com.* June 5, 2013. http://www.cnn.com/2013/06/04/politics/chambliss-sexual-assaults.

Garrison, William Lloyd. "The Relation of Poverty to Purity." In *The National Purity Congress*, edited by Aaron M. Powell, 398–405. New York: American Purity Alliance, 1896.

Gay, Joseph R. *Life Lines of Success: A Practical Manual of Self Help for the Future Development of the Ambitious Colored American.* Chicago: W. R. Vansant, 1913.

Ghee, Peter F. "Chronic Gonorrhoea." *Journal of the National Medical Association* 2, no. 2 (1910): 79.

Gibson, J. W., Mrs. J. W. Gibson, and W. J. Truitt. *Golden Thoughts on Chastity and Procreation.* Naperville, IL: J. L. Nichols, 1903.

———. *Social Purity, or, the Life of the Home and Nation.* Naperville, IL: J. L. Nichols, 1903.

Girl Scouts of the USA. *Scouting for Girls: Official Handbook of the Girl Scouts.* 1st ed. New York: Girl Scouts, 1920.

Goldman, Emma. *Living My Life.* New York: Alfred A. Knopf, 1931.

Griggs, Edward Howard. *Moral Education.* Croton-on-Hudson: Orchard Hill Press, 1903.

Gulick, Luther. "Boys' and Girls' Organizations and Social Hygiene." *Journal of the Society of Sanitary and Moral Prophylaxis* 5 (1914): 181–91.

———. *Morals and Morale.* New York: Association Press, 1919.

Hackley, E. Azalia. *The Colored Girl Beautiful.* Kansas City, MO: Burton, 1916.

Haeckel, Ernst. *The Riddle of the Universe at the Close of the Nineteenth Century*. Translated by Joseph McCabe. New York: Harper, 1900.

Hall, G. Stanley. *Adolescence: Its Psychology and Its Relations to Physiology, Anthropology, Sociology, Sex, Crime, Religion, and Education*. 2 vols. New York: Appleton, 1904.

———. "Sex Hygiene in Infantile and Pre-pubertal Life." In *Transactions of the Fourth International Congress on School Hygiene*. Buffalo, NY, 1913.

Hall, Josie Briggs. *Hall's Moral and Mental Capsule for the Economic and Domestic Life of the Negro, as a Solution of the Race Problem*. Dallas: R. S. Jenkins, 1905.

Hall, Radclyffe. *The Well of Loneliness*. London: Jonathan Cape, 1928.

Hall, Winfield Scott. *The Biology, Physiology and Sociology of Reproduction, Also Sexual Hygiene, with Special Reference to the Male*. Chicago: Wynnewood, 1907.

———. *Daughter, Mother and Father: A Story for Girls*. Chicago: AMA Press, 1913.

A Handbook for Leaders of Younger Girls. Girls' Work Series. New York: Young Women's Christian Association, 1919.

H. E. K. "Sex Hygiene Exhibit for Recruits at Jefferson Barracks." *Texas State Journal of Medicine* 13 (1917): 191.

Hensley, Scott. "Pediatricians Fact-Check Bachmann's Bashing of HPV Vaccine." *NPR.org*. September 13, 2011. http://www.npr.org/blogs/ health/2011/09/ 13/140445104/pediatricians-fact-check-bachmanns-bashing-of-hpv-vaccine.

Hetherington, Clark W. "Play Leadership in Sex Education." *Journal of Social Hygiene* 1, no. 1 (1914): 36–43.

Home Reading Course for Citizen-Soldiers. War Information Series 9. Washington, DC: Committee on Public Information, 1917.

Hooker, Edith Houghton. "A Criticism of Venereal Prophylaxis." *Journal of Social Hygiene* 4, no. 2 (1918): 179–95.

Howard, William Lee. "The Negro as a Distinct Ethnic Factor in Civilization." *Medicine* 60 (1903): 423–26.

Hoxie, W. J. *How Girls Can Help Their Country*. Bedford, MA: Applewood Books, 1913.

Hunton, Addie W., and Kathryn M. Johnson. *Two Colored Women with the American Expeditionary Forces*. Brooklyn: Brooklyn Eagle Press, 1920.

"An Interesting Book on the Negro." *Southern Medical Journal* 8, no. 4 (1915): 337.

Johnson, William. "'Regulation' in the Philippines." *Woman's Journal*, November 10, 1900, 356.

Joyce, Thomas Athol. "Negro." In *All There Is to Know: Readings from the Illustrious Eleventh Edition of the Encyclopedia Britannica*, edited by Charles Simmons, 245–46. New York: Simon and Schuster, 1910.

Kenney, John A. "Eugenics and the School Teacher." *Journal of the National Medical Association* 7, no. 4 (1915): 253–54.

———. "Salutatory." *Journal of the National Medical Association* 1, no. 2 (1909): 38.

———. "Syphilis and the American Negro—a Medico-Sociologic Study." *Journal of the National Medical Association* 1, no. 2 (1909): 115–17.

Keyes, E. L. "Personals." *Survey*, April 12, 1913, 76.

Kliff, Sarah. "Rep. Todd Akin Is Wrong about Rape and Pregnancy, but He's Not Alone," *Washington Post Online*, August 20, 2012. http://www.washingtonpost.com/ blogs/wonkblog/wp/2012/08/20/rep-todd-akin-is-wrong-about-rape-and-pregnancy-but-hes-not-alone/.

Knebel, Aaron G. *Four Decades with Men and Boys.* New York: Association Press, 1936.

Knowlton, Charles. *Fruits of Philosophy, or the Private Companion of Adult People.* Philadelphia: F. P. Rogers, 1839.

Lashley, Karl S., and John B. Watson. "A Psychological Study of Motion Pictures in Relation to Venereal Disease Campaigns." *Social Hygiene* 7, no. 2 (1921): 181–219.

"Law Enforcement Notes." *Social Hygiene Bulletin* 5, no. 4 (1918): 8.

"Lay Familiarity with 606." *Journal of the National Medical Association* 3, no. 2 (1911): 126.

Lee, William Howard. "The Negro as a Distinct Ethnic Factor in Civilization." *Medicine* 60 (1903): 423–26.

"Legal Protection for Young Girls." *Philanthropist* 1, no. 1 (1886): 4–5.

Lewis, Denslow. *The Gynecologic Consideration of the Sexual Act.* Chicago: Henry O. Shepard, 1900.

Lynch, Kenneth M., Kater McInnes, and G. Fleming McInnes. "Concerning Syphilis in the American Negro." *Southern Medical Journal* 8, no. 6 (1915): 450–56.

Lyttleton, Edward. "Instructions in Matters of Sex." *Educational Review* 46 (1913): 135–42.

McCulloch, James, ed. *Democracy in Earnest.* New York: Negro Universities Press, 1918.

McHatton, Henry. "The Sexual Status of the Negro—Past and Present." *American Journal of Dermatology and Genito-Urinary Diseases* 10, no. 1 (1906): 6–9.

"Medical Declaration Concerning Chastity." *Philanthropist* 10, no. 1 (1895): 5.

Moore, H. C. "Report on the Committee on Study of Venereal Diseases." *Texas State Journal of Medicine* 12 (1917): 419.

Moore, Joanna P. *"In Christ's Stead": Autobiographical Sketches.* Chicago: Women's Baptist Home Mission Society, 1902.

Morrow, Prince A. "The Prophylaxis of Venereal Diseases: Medical Aspects of the Social Evil in New York." *Philadelphia Medical Journal* 7 (1901): 663–69.

———. *Publicity as a Factor in Venereal Prophylaxis.* Chicago: Press of the American Medical Association, 1906.

———. *Social Diseases and Marriage.* New York: Lea Brothers, 1904.

Mosher, Clelia Duel. *Health and the Woman Movement.* New York: Young Women's Christian Association, 1916.

———. *The Mosher Survey: Sexual Attitudes of 45 Victorian Women.* New York: Arno Press, 1980.

Murrell, Thomas W. "Syphilis and the American Negro." *Journal of the American Medical Association* 54, no. 11 (1910): 847.

"The National Health Week for Negroes." Editorial. *Southern Medical Journal* 8, no. 8 (1915): 734.

"The Negro as a Factor in the Work of Preventive Medicine in the South." *Southern Medical Journal* 1, no. 6 (1908): 390.

"The New Game of Playing with Fire and the Right Not to Be Forced to Know Evil." *Century*, March 1913, 795–96.

"News." *Texas State Journal of Medicine* 15 (August 1919): 163.

Oberholtzer, Ellis Paxon. *The Morals of the Movies.* Philadelphia: Penn, 1922.

Odum, Howard W. *Social and Mental Traits of the Negro: Research into the Conditions of the Negro Race in Southern Towns.* New York: Columbia University Press, 1910.

Owen, Robert Dale. *Moral Physiology, or a Brief and Plain Treatise on the Population Question.* New York: G. Vale, 1830.

"A Phase of Birth Control." *Journal of the National Medical Association* 12, no. 1 (1920): 31.

Phelan, James D. "The Japanese Evil in California," *North American Review* 21, no. 762 (September 1919): 323–28.

"Physician to Lecture to Soldiers Stationed at Fort Worth." *Texas State Journal of Medicine* 13 (1917): 193.

Post, George W. *The Cottage Physician: For Individual and Family Use.* Springfield: King-Richardson, 1897.

Powdermaker, Hortense. *After Freedom: A Cultural Study in the Deep South.* New York: Viking Press, 1939.

Powell, Aaron M., ed. *The National Purity Congress: Its Papers, Addresses, Portraits.* New York: American Purity Alliance, 1896.

Powell, Anna Rice. "The Moral Elevation of Girls." *Philanthropist* 1, no. 2 (1886): 3.

"Prospects in the South." *American Social Hygiene Association Bulletin* 1, no. 3 (1914): 1.

Quillian, Daniel David. "Racial Peculiarities: A Cause of the Prevalence of Syphilis in Negroes." *American Journal of Dermatology and Genito-Urinary Diseases* 10 (1906): 277–79.

Reynolds, Jason Bronson. "The Union of the American Vigilance Association and the American Federation for Sex Hygiene." *Vigilance* 27, no. 10 (1913): 1.

Rhetta, Barnett M. "A Plea for the Lives of the Unborn." *Journal of the National Medical Association* 7, no. 3 (1915): 200–205.

Rippin, Jane Deeter. "Social Hygiene and the War." *Journal of Social Hygiene* 5 (1919): 125–36.

Robie, Walter Franklin. *Sex Histories: Authentic Sex Experiences of Men and Women Showing How Fear and Ignorance of the Sex Life Lead to Individual Misery and Social Depravity.* London: Amalgamated Medical Press, 1922.

Robinson, William J. *Sex Knowledge for Men Including a Program for Sex Education of the Boy.* New York: Critic and Guide, 1916.

Roman, Charles V. *American Civilization and the Negro: The Afro-American in Relation to National Progress.* Philadelphia: F. A. Davis, 1916.

———. "The Negro Woman and the Health Problem." *Journal of the National Medical Association* 7, no. 3 (1915): 185.

———. "Some Ramifications of the Sexual Impulse." *Journal of the National Medical Association* 12, no. 1 (1920): 14–17.

Roosevelt, Theodore. *The Strenuous Life: Essays and Addresses.* New York: Century, 1901.

Sanger, Margaret. *Family Limitation.* New York: 1914.

———. *Margaret Sanger: An Autobiography.* New York: W. W. Norton, 1938.

———. "No Gods No Masters." *Woman Rebel* 1, no. 1 (1914): 1, 8, 16.

———. *What Every Girl Should Know.* New York: M. N. Maisel, 1920.

———. *Woman and the New Race.* New York: Truth, 1920.

Sawyer, Wilbur A. "Venereal Disease Control in the Military Forces." *American Journal of Public Health* 9, no. 5 (1919): 337–45.

"Sex Hygiene Lectures Given to Boy Scouts." *Scouting* 1, no. 10 (1913): 8.

"Sex Topics in the Schools." *Journal of Education*, November 27, 1913, 538.

Seymour, Gertrude. "The Health of Soldier and Civilian." *Survey*, April 24, 1918, 89–94.

Shepley Sergent, Elizabeth. "The Temper of the A. E. F." *New Republic*, July 20, 1918, 336–38.

"606." *Journal of the National Medical Association* 3, no. 1 (1911): 63.

Smith, Fred B. "Four Sins That Soldiers Say They Hate." *American Magazine*, November 1918, 12–13, 129–33.

Snow, William F. "Progress: 1900–1915." In *American Social Hygiene Association*, 40–41. Minneapolis, 1915.

Snow, William F., and Wilbur A. Sawyer. "Venereal Disease Control in the Army." *Journal of the American Medical Association* 71, no. 6 (1918): 456–63.

Spingarn, Arthur B. "The War and Venereal Diseases among Negroes." *Journal of Social Hygiene* 4, no. 3 (1918): 333–46.

Stockham, Alice B. *Tokology: A Book for Every Woman*. 1894 ed. Chicago: Alice B. Stockham, 1887. First published 1893 by R. F. Fenno.

Tierney, Richard H. "The Catholic Church and the Sex Problem." *Journal of Education*, September 25, 1913, 285–86.

Turner, Dr. "Vice Disease, Our Social and Economic Peril." *Journal of the National Medical Association* 5, no. 4 (1913): 250.

United States Public Health Service. *Annual Report of the Surgeon General of the Public Health Service of the United States*. Washington, DC: Government Printing Office, 1921.

Vedder, Edward Bright. *Syphilis and Public Health*. Philadelphia: Lea & Febiger, 1918.

Walker, George. *Venereal Disease in the American Expeditionary Forces*. Baltimore: Medical Standard Book, 1922.

Warden, Randall D. "Why Give Sex Instruction in High Schools." *Transactions of the Fourth International Congress on School Hygiene* 3 (1913): 180.

War Department. *Annual Report of the Secretary of War for the Fiscal Year, 1918*. Vol. 1 (Washington DC: Government Printing Office, 1918).

Willard, Frances E. "Frances E. Willard on Social Purity." *Philanthropist* 1, no. 1 (1886): 2.

Willson, Robert. "An Outline Program for the Teaching of Sex Hygiene in the Schools." In *Transactions of the Fourth International Conference on School Hygiene*, 3:29–37. Buffalo, NY, 1913.

Woodson, Carter G. *The Mis-education of the Negro*. Washington: Associated, 1933.

Secondary Sources

Adas, Michael. *Machines as the Measure of Men: Science, Technology, and Ideologies of Western Dominance*. Ithaca: Cornell University Press, 1989.

African American Registry. "Black History and the Girl Scouts of America." Accessed November 25, 2014. http://www.aaregistry.org/historic_events/view/black-history-and-girl-scouts-america.

Alexander, Eleanor. *Lyrics of Sunshine and Shadow: The Tragic Courtship and Marriage of Paul Laurence Dunbar and Alice Ruth Moore.* New York: New York University Press, 2001.

Alonso, Harriet Hyman. *Peace as a Women's Issue: A History of the U.S. Movement for World Peace and Women's Rights.* Syracuse, NY: Syracuse University Press, 1993.

American Film Institute. Catalog of Silent Films. Accessed April 7, 2005. http://www.afi.com/members/catalog/silentHome.aspx?s=1.

Anderson, Ann. *Snake Oil, Hustlers and Hambones: The American Medicine Show.* Jefferson, NC: McFarland, 2000.

Apple, Rima D. *Mothers and Medicine: A Social History of Infant Feeding, 1890–1950.* Madison: University of Wisconsin Press, 1987.

————, ed. *Women, Health, and Medicine in America: A Historical Handbook.* New York: Garland, 1990.

Arnold, David. *Colonizing the Body: State Medicine and Epidemic Disease in Nineteenth-Century India.* Berkeley: University of California Press, 1993.

Ayers, Edward L. *The Promise of the New South: Life after Reconstruction.* New York: Oxford University Press, 1992.

Bailey, Beth. *From Front Porch to Back Seat: Courtship in Twentieth-Century America.* Baltimore: Johns Hopkins University Press, 1988.

Baker, Jean H. *Margaret Sanger: A Life of Passion.* New York: Hill and Wang, 2011.

Barbeau, Arthur E., and Florette Henri. *The Unknown Soldiers, African-American Troops in World War I.* Philadelphia: Temple University Press, 1974.

Bashford, Alison, and Carolyn Strange. "Public Pedagogy: Sex Education and Mass Communication in the Mid-twentieth Century." *Journal of the History of Sexuality* 13, no. 1 (2004): 71–99.

Bederman, Gail. *Manliness and Civilization: A Cultural History of Gender and Race in the United States, 1880–1917.* Chicago: University of Chicago Press, 1995.

Behr, Edward. *Prohibition: Thirteen Years That Changed America.* New York: Arcade, 1996.

Belkin, Aaron. *Bring Me Men: Military Masculinity and the Benign Façade of American Empire, 1898–2001.* New York: Columbia University Press, 2012.

Black, Gregory D. *Hollywood Censored: Morality Codes, Catholics, and the Movies.* Cambridge: Cambridge University Press, 1994.

Brandt, Allan M. *No Magic Bullet: A Social History of Venereal Disease in the United States since 1880.* New York: Oxford University Press, 1985.

Briggs, Laura. "The Race of Hysteria: 'Overcivilization' and the 'Savage' Woman in Late Nineteenth-Century Obstetrics and Gynecology." *American Quarterly* 52, no. 2 (2000): 246–73.

Bristow, Nancy K. *Making Men Moral: Social Engineering during the Great War.* New York: New York University Press, 1996.

Brumberg, Joan Jacobs. *The Body Project: An Intimate History of American Girls.* New York: Random House, 1997.

————. "'Something Happens to Girls': Menarche and the Emergence of the Modern American Hygiene Imperative." *Journal of the History of Sexuality* 4, no. 1 (1993): 99–127.

Buckler, Helen, Mary Fielder, and Martha Allen. *Wo-He-Lo: The Story of the Camp Fire Girls 1910–1960.* New York: Holt, Rinehart & Winston, 1961.

Burnham, John C. "The Progressive Era Revolution in American Attitudes toward Sex." *Journal of American History* 59, no. 4 (1973): 885–908.

Burrow, James G. *Organized Medicine in the Progressive Era.* Baltimore: Johns Hopkins University Press, 1977.

———. *AMA: Voice of American Medicine.* Baltimore: Johns Hopkins Press, 1963.

Butchart, Alexander. *The Anatomy of Power: European Constructions of the African Body.* London: Zed Books, 1998.

Campbell, Patricia J. *Sex Guides: Books and Films about Sexuality for Young Adults.* New York: Garland, 1986.

Canaday, Margot. *The Straight State: Sexuality and Citizenship in Twentieth-Century America.* Princeton, NJ: Princeton University Press, 2009.

Carstens, Lisa. "Unbecoming Women: Sex Reversal in the Scientific Discourse on Female Deviance in Britain, 1880–1920." *Journal of the History of Sexuality* 20, no. 1 (2011): 62–95.

Carter, Julian B. "Birds, Bees, and Venereal Disease: Toward an Intellectual History of Sex Education." *Journal of the History of Sexuality* 10, no. 2 (2001): 213–49.

———. *The Heart of Whiteness: Normal Sexuality and Race in America, 1880–1940.* Durham, NC: Duke University Press, 2010.

Chapman, Erin D. *Prove It on Me: New Negroes, Sex, and Popular Culture in the 1920s.* New York: Oxford University Press, 2012.

Charatz-Litt, Cynthia. "A Chronicle of Racism: The Effects of the White Medical Community on Black Health." *Journal of the National Medical Association* 84, no. 8 (1992): 717–25.

Chauncey, George. "Christian Brotherhood or Sexual Perversion? Homosexual Identities and the Construction of Sexual Boundaries in the World War One Era." *Journal of Social History* 19 (1985): 189–211.

———. *Gay New York: Gender, Urban Culture, and the Making of the Gay Male World, 1890–1940.* New York: Basic Books, 1994.

Chen, Constance. *The Sex Side of Life: Mary Ware Dennett's Pioneering Battle for Birth Control and Sex Education.* New York: New Press, 1996.

Chesler, Ellen. *Woman of Valor: Margaret Sanger and the Birth Control Movement in America.* New York: Simon and Schuster, 1992.

Christian, Garna L. "Newton Baker's War on El Paso Vice." *Red River Valley Historical Review* 5, no. 2 (1980): 55–67.

Clarke, Walter. "Dr. Prince Albert Morrow and His Aides." *Journal of Social Hygiene* 40, no. 5 (1954): 181–94.

Coffman, Edward M. *The War to End All Wars. The American Military Experience in World War I.* New York: Oxford University Press, 1968.

Connelly, Mark Thomas. *The Response to Prostitution in the Progressive Era.* Chapel Hill: University of North Carolina Press, 1980.

Cook, James R. "The Evolution of Sex Education in the Public Schools of the United States, 1900–1970." PhD diss., Southern Illinois University, 1971.

Cordasco, Francesco, and Thomas Monroe Pitkin. *The White Slave Trade and the Immigrants: A Chapter in American Social History.* Detroit: Blaine Ethridge, 1981.

Cornog, Martha. *For Sex Education, See Librarian: A Guide to Issues and Resources.* New York: Greenwood Press, 1996.

Cott, Nancy. *The Bonds of Womanhood: "Woman's Sphere" in New England, 1780–1835*. New Haven, CT: Yale University Press, 1977.

———. *The Grounding of Modern Feminism*. New Haven, CT: Yale University Press, 1987.

———. "Passionlessness: An Interpretation of Victorian Sexual Ideology, 1790–1850." *Signs: Journal of Women in Culture and Society* 4, no. 2 (1978): 219–36.

Cremin, Lawrence. *American Education: The Metropolitan Experience, 1876–1980*. New York: Harper and Row, 1988.

———. *The Transformation of the School: Progressivism in American Education, 1876–1957*. New York: Alfred A. Knopf, 1961.

Curwood, Anastasia. *Stormy Weather: Middle-Class African American Marriages between the Two World Wars*. Chapel Hill: University of North Carolina Press, 2010.

Dailey, Jane. "The Theology of Massive Resistance: Sex, Segregation, and the Sacred after *Brown*." In *Massive Resistance: Southern Opposition to the Second Reconstruction*, edited by Clive Webb, 151–80. Oxford: Oxford University Press, 2005.

Daniels, Jonathan. *The End of Innocence*. New York: Da Capo Press, 1972.

Davies, Mel. "Corsets and Conception: Fashion and Demographic Trends in the Nineteenth Century." *Comparative Studies in Society and History* 24, no. 4 (1982): 611–41.

Delany, Sarah, A. Elizabeth Delany, and Amy Hill Hearth. *Having Our Say: The Delany Sisters' First 100 Years*. New York: Dell, 1993.

De Leon, Arnoldo. *They Called Them Greasers: Anglo Attitudes toward Mexicans in Texas, 1821–1900*. Austin: University of Texas Press, 1983.

D'Emilio, John, and Estelle Freedman. *Intimate Matters: A History of Sexuality in America*. New York: Harper and Row, 1988.

DeRogatis, Amy. "What Would Jesus Do? Sexuality and Salvation in Protestant Evangelical Sex Manuals, 1950s to the Present." *Church History* 74, no. 1 (2005): 97–137.

Donovan, Brian. *White Slave Crusades: Race, Gender, and Anti-vice Activism, 1887–1917*. Urbana: University of Illinois Press, 2006.

Duberman, Martin Bauml, Martha Vicinus, and George Chauncey Jr. *Hidden from History: Reclaiming the Gay and Lesbian Past*. New York: New American Library, 1989.

Dunlap, Leslie K. "The Reform of Rape Law and the Problem of White Men: Age-of-Consent Campaigns in the South, 1885–1910." In *Sex, Love, Race: Crossing Boundaries in North American History*, edited by Martha Hodes, 352–72. New York: New York University Press, 1999.

Dyer, Thomas G. *Theodore Roosevelt and the Idea of Race*. Baton Rouge: Louisiana State University Press, 1980.

Eberwein, Robert. *Sex Ed: Film, Video, and the Framework of Desire*. New Brunswick, NJ: Rutgers University Press, 1999.

Engelstein, Laura. "Morality and the Wooden Spoon: Russian Doctors View Syphilis, Social Class, and Sexual Behavior, 1890–1905." In *The Making of the Modern Body: Sexuality and Society in the Nineteenth Century*, edited by Thomas Walter Laqueur, 169–208. Berkeley: University of California Press, 1987.

Etheridge, Elizabeth W. *The Butterfly Caste: A Social History of Pellagra in the South*. Westport, CT: Greenwood Press, 1972.

Ettling, John. *The Germ of Laziness: Rockefeller Philanthropy and Public Health in the New South*. Cambridge, MA: Harvard University Press, 1981.

Evans, Sara. *Born for Liberty: A History of Women in America*. New York: Free Press, 1989.

Faderman, Lillian. *Odd Girls and Twilight Lovers: A History of Lesbian Life in Twentieth-Century America*. New York: Columbia University Press, 1991.

———. *Surpassing the Love of Men: Romantic Friendship and Love between Women from the Renaissance to the Present*. New York: William Morrow, 1981.

Fass, Paula. *The Damned and the Beautiful: American Youth in the 1920s*. New York: Oxford University Press, 1977.

Fett, Sharla M. *Working Cures: Healing, Health and Power on Southern Slave Plantations*. Chapel Hill: University of North Carolina Press, 2002.

Filene, Peter G. *Him/Her/Self: Sex Roles in Modern America*. New York: Harcourt Brace Jovanovich, 1975.

Findlay, Eileen. *Imposing Decency: The Politics of Sexuality and Race in Puerto Rico, 1870–1920*. Durham, NC: Duke University Press, 1999.

Fogel, Robert William, and Stanley Engerman. *Time on the Cross: The Economics of American Negro Slavery*. Boston: Little, Brown, 1974.

Foley, Neil. "Partly Colored or Other White: Mexican Americans and Their Problems with the Color Line." In *Beyond Black and White: Race, Ethnicity, and Gender in the U.S. South and Southwest*, edited by Stephanie Cole and Alison M. Parker, 123–44. College Station: Texas A&M University Press, 2004.

———. *The White Scourge: Mexicans, Blacks, and Poor Whites in Texas Cotton Culture*. Berkeley: University of California Press, 1997.

Fosdick, Raymond B. *Chronicle of a Generation: An Autobiography*. New York: Harper and Brothers, 1958.

———. "Fit for Fighting—and After." *Scribner's*, April 1918, 415–23. Also available in 1919, folder 131:2, ASHA Papers.

Foucault, Michel. *The History of Sexuality*. Vol. 1, *An Introduction*. Translated by Robert Hurley. New York: Pantheon Books, 1976.

Frazier, E. Franklin. *The Negro Church in America*. New York: Schocken Books, 1963.

Freedman, Estelle. "Sexuality in Nineteenth-Century America: Behavior, Ideology, and Politics." *Reviews in American History* 10 (December 1982): 196–215.

Freeman, Susan K. *Sex Goes to School: Girls and Sex Education Before the 1960s*. Urbana: University of Illinois Press, 2008.

Frisken, Amanda. *Victoria Woodhull's Sexual Revolution: Political Theater and the Popular Press in Nineteenth-Century America*. Philadelphia: University of Pennsylvania Press, 2004.

Gabbert, Ann R. "Prostitution and Moral Reform in the Borderlands: El Paso, 1890–1920." *Journal of the History of Sexuality* 12, no. 4 (2003): 575–604.

Gaines, Kevin K. *Uplifting the Race: Black Leadership, Politics, and Culture in the Twentieth Century*. Chapel Hill: University of North Carolina Press, 1996.

Gatewood, Willard B. *Aristocrats of Color: The Black Elite, 1880–1920*. Bloomington: Indiana University Press, 1990.

Giddings, Paula. *Where and When I Enter: The Impact of Black Women on Race and Sex in America*. New York: William Morrow, 1984.

Gilman, Sander L. *Difference and Pathology: Stereotypes of Sexuality, Race, and Madness.* Ithaca, NY: Cornell University Press, 1985.

Gilmore, Glenda Elizabeth. *Gender and Jim Crow: Women and the Politics of White Supremacy in North Carolina, 1896–1920.* Chapel Hill: University of North Carolina Press, 1996.

Glenn, Evelyn Nakano. *Unequal Freedom: How Race and Gender Shaped American Citizenship and Labor.* Cambridge, MA: Harvard University Press, 2002.

Gordon, Linda. *Pitied but Not Entitled: Single Mothers and the History of Welfare, 1890–1935.* New York: Free Press, 1994.

———. *Woman's Body, Woman's Right: A Social History of Birth Control in America.* New York: Grossman, 1976.

Gutman, Herbert. *The Black Family in Slavery and Freedom, 1750–1925.* New York: Vintage Books, 1976.

———. *Slavery and the Numbers Game: A Critique of "Time on the Cross."* Urbana: University of Illinois Press, 1975.

Guy-Sheftall, Beverly. "Sinner or Saint? Antithetical Views concerning Black Women and the Private Sphere." In *Daughters of Sorrow: Black Women in United States History,* 37–90. Brooklyn: Carlson, 1990.

Hall, Jacquelyn Dowd. *Revolt against Chivalry: Jessie Daniel Ames and the Women's Campaign against Lynching.* New York: Columbia University Press, 1979.

Haller, John S. *Outcasts from Evolution: Scientific Attitudes of Racial Inferiority, 1859–1900.* Urbana: University of Illinois Press, 1971.

Haller, John S., and Robin Haller. *The Physician and Sexuality in Victorian America.* Rev. ed. Carbondale: Southern Illinois University Press, 1995.

Haller, Mark. *Eugenics: Hereditarian Attitudes in American Thought.* New Brunswick, NJ: Rutgers University Press, 1963.

Harr, John Ensor, and Peter J. Johnson. *The Rockefeller Century.* New York: Scribner's, 1988.

Harrison, Mark. "The Tender Frame of Man: Disease, Climate, and Racial Difference in India and the West Indies, 1760–1860." *Bulletin of the History of Medicine* 70, no. 1 (1996): 68–93.

Harsin, Jill. "Syphilis, Wives, and Physicians: Medical Ethics and the Family in Late Nineteenth-Century Paris." *French Historical Studies* 16, no. 1 (1989): 72–95.

Hart, Jamie. "Who Should Have the Children? Discussions of Birth Control among African-American Intellectuals, 1920–1939." *Journal of Negro History* 79, no. 1 (1994): 71–84.

Hicks, Cheryl. *Talk with You Like a Woman: African American Women, Justice, and Reform in New York, 1890–1935.* Chapel Hill: University of North Carolina Press, 2010.

Higginbotham, Evelyn Brooks. *Righteous Discontent: The Women's Movement in the Black Baptist Church, 1880–1920.* Cambridge, MA: Harvard University Press, 1993.

Higham, John. *Strangers in the Land: Patterns of American Nativism, 1860–1925.* New Brunswick, NJ: Rutgers University Press, 1955.

Hine, Darlene Clark. "Rape and the Inner Lives of Black Women in the Middle West: Preliminary Thoughts on the Culture of Dissemblance." *Signs: Journal of Women in Culture and Society* 14, no. 4 (1988): 912–20.

Hobson, Barbara Meil. *Uneasy Virtue: The Politics of Prostitution and the American Reform Tradition.* New York: Basic Books, 1987.

Howe, Daniel Walker. "American Victorianism as a Culture." *American Quarterly* 27, no. 5 (1975): 507–32.

Hunter, Jane H. *How Young Ladies Became Girls: The Victorian Origins of American Girlhood.* New Haven, CT: Yale University Press, 2002.

Hunter, Tera. *To 'Joy My Freedom: Southern Black Women's Lives and Labors after the Civil War.* Cambridge, MA: Harvard University Press, 1997.

Imber, Michael. "Analysis of a Curriculum Reform Movement: The American Social Hygiene Association's Campaign for Sex Education, 1900–1930." PhD diss., Stanford University, 1980.

———. "The First World War, Sex Education, and the American Social Hygiene Association's Campaign against Venereal Disease." *Journal of Educational Administration and History* 16, no. 1 (1984): 47–56.

———. "Toward a Theory of Curriculum Reform: An Analysis of the First Campaign for Sex Education." *Curriculum Inquiry* 12, no. 4 (1982): 339–62.

Irons, Peter. *Jim Crow's Children: The Broken Promise of the Brown Decision.* New York: Viking Penguin, 2002.

Irvine, Janice. *Talk about Sex: The Battle over Sex Education in the United States.* Berkeley: University of California Press, 2004.

Jacobson, Matthew Frye. *Barbarian Virtues: The United States Encounters Foreign Peoples at Home and Abroad, 1876–1917.* New York: Hill and Wang, 2000.

———. *Whiteness of a Different Color: European Immigrants and the Alchemy of Race.* Cambridge, MA: Harvard University Press, 1998.

Jensen, Kimberly. *Mobilizing Minerva: American Women in the First World War.* Urbana: University of Illinois Press, 2008.

———. "'Venereal Girls,' the Cedars Detention Home, and the Portland Free Dispensary." OHSU History of Medicine Society Lecture Series, October 18, 2013.

Jones, James. *Alfred C. Kinsey: A Life.* New York: W. W. Norton, 1997.

———. *Bad Blood: The Tuskegee Syphilis Experiment.* New York: Free Press, 1981.

Kaestle, Carl F. *Pillars of the Republic: Common Schools and American Society 1780–1860.* New York: Hill and Wang, 1983.

Kennedy, David. *Over Here: The First World War and American Society.* New York: Oxford University Press, 1980.

Kennedy, Kathleen. *Disloyal Mothers and Scurrilous Citizens: Women and Subversion during World War I.* Bloomington: Indiana University Press, 1999.

Kerber, Linda K. *No Constitutional Right to Be Ladies: Women and the Obligations of Citizenship.* New York: Hill and Wang, 1998.

Kern, Louis. *An Ordered Love: Sex Roles and Sexuality in Victorian Utopias: The Shakers, the Mormons, and the Oneida Community.* Chapel Hill: University of North Carolina Press, 1981.

Kett, Joseph F. *Rites of Passage: Adolescence in America, 1790 to the Present.* New York: Basic Books, 1977.

Kevles, Daniel. *In the Name of Eugenics: Genetics and the Uses of Human Heredity.* New York: Knopf, 1985.

Kirby, Jack Temple. *Darkness at the Dawning: Race and Reform in the Progressive South.* Philadelphia: Lippincott, 1972.

Kish Sklar, Kathryn. *Florence Kelley and the Nation's Work: The Rise of Women's Political Culture, 1830–1900.* New Haven, CT: Yale University Press, 1995.

Kohler, Pamale K., Lisa E. Manhart, William T. Lafferty. "Abstinence-Only and Comprehensive Sex Education and the Initiation of Sexual Activity and Teen Pregnancy." *Journal of Adolescent Health* 42, no. 4 (April 2008): 344–51.

Kolchin, Peter. "Whiteness Studies: The New History of Race in America." *Journal of American History* 89, no. 1 (2002): 154–73.

Koslow, Jennifer Lisa. *Cultivating Health: Los Angeles Women and Public Health Reform.* New Brunswick, NJ: Rutgers University Press, 2009.

Kraditor, Aileen S. *The Ideas of the Woman Suffrage Movement, 1890–1920.* New York: Columbia University Press, 1965.

Kuhn, Annette. *Cinema, Censorship and Sexuality, 1909–1925.* London: Routledge, 1988.

Larson, Edward. *Sex, Race, and Science: Eugenics in the Deep South.* Baltimore: Johns Hopkins University Press, 1995.

Lasch-Quinn, Elisabeth. *Black Neighbors: Race and the Limits of Reform in the American Settlement House Movement, 1890–1945.* Chapel Hill: University of North Carolina Press, 1993.

Lawrence, Leonard E. "Why the NMA: Its Heritage Revisited and Future Challenges Assessed." *Journal of the National Medical Association* 85, no. 10 (1993): 745–48.

Lederhendler, Eli. *Jewish Responses to Modernity: New Voices in America and Eastern Europe.* New York: New York University Press, 1994.

Lee, Ulysses. *The Employment of Negro Troops.* Washington, DC: Government Printing Office, 2000.

Lewis, David Levering. *When Harlem Was in Vogue.* New York: Oxford University Press, 1979.

Limón, José E. "Tex-Sex-Mex: American Identities, Lone Stars, and the Politics of Racialized Sexuality." *American Literary History* 9, no. 3 (1997): 598–616.

Link, William A. *The Paradox of Southern Progressivism, 1880–1930.* Chapel Hill: University of North Carolina Press, 1992.

Lissak, Rivka Shpak. *Pluralism and Progressives: Hull House and the New Immigrants, 1890–1919.* Chicago: University of Chicago Press, 1989.

Long, Alecia P. *The Great Southern Babylon: Sex, Race, and Respectability in New Orleans, 1865–1920.* Baton Rouge: Louisiana State University Press, 2004.

Lord, Alexandra M. *Condom Nation: The U.S. Government's Sex Education Campaign from World War I to the Internet.* Baltimore: Johns Hopkins University Press, 2009.

———. "Models of Masculinity: Sex Education, the United States Public Health Service, and the YMCA, 1919–1924." *Journal of the History of Medicine and Allied Sciences* 58, no. 2 (2003): 123–52.

———. "'Naturally Clean and Wholesome': Women, Sex Education, and the United States Public Health Service, 1918–1928." *Social History of Medicine* 17, no. 3 (2004): 423–41.

Lunbeck, Elizabeth. "'A New Generation of Women': Progressive Psychiatrists and the Hypersexual Female." *Feminist Studies* 13 (Autumn 1987): 513–43.

MacDonald, Robert H. *Sons of the Empire: The Frontier and the Boy Scout Movement.* Toronto: University of Toronto Press, 1993.

Macleod, David I. *Building Character in the American Boy: The Boy Scouts, YMCA, and Their Forerunners, 1870–1920.* Madison: University of Wisconsin Press, 1983.

Martin, Emily. *The Woman in the Body: A Cultural Analysis of Reproduction.* Boston: Beacon Press, 1987.

Maw, Wallace. "Fifty Years of Sex Education in the Public Schools of the United States (1900–1950): A History of Ideas." PhD diss., University of Cincinnati, 1953.

Mayer, Holly A. *Belonging to the Army: Camp Followers and Community during the American Revolution.* Columbia: University of South Carolina Press, 1996.

McGirr, Lisa. *Suburban Warriors: The Origins of the New American Right.* Princeton, NJ: Princeton University Press, 2001.

McGuire, Danielle. *At the Dark End of the Street: Black Women, Rape, and Resistance—a New History of the Civil Rights Movement from Rosa Parks to the Rise of Black Power.* New York: Knopf, 2010.

Mechling, Jay. *On My Honor: Boy Scouts and the Making of American Youth.* Chicago: University of Chicago Press, 2001.

Melody, Michael Edward, and Linda Mary Peterson. *Teaching America about Sex: Marriage Guides and Sex Manuals from the Late Victorians to Dr. Ruth.* New York: New York University Press, 1999.

Miller, Susan A. "Girls in Nature / the Nature of Girls: Transforming Female Adolescence at Summer Camp, 1900–1939." PhD diss., University of Pennsylvania, 2001.

Mintz, Steven. *Huck's Raft: A History of American Childhood.* Cambridge, MA: Belknap Press, 2004.

Mitchell, Michele. *Righteous Propagation: African Americans and the Politics of Racial Destiny after Reconstruction.* Chapel Hill: University of North Carolina Press, 2004.

Mitchell, Pablo. *West of Sex: Making Mexican America, 1900–1930.* Chicago: University of Chicago Press, 2012.

Mjagkij, Nina. *Light in the Darkness: African Americans and the YMCA, 1852–1946.* Lexington: University of Kentucky Press, 1994.

Molina, Natalia. *Fit to Be Citizens? Public Health and Race in Los Angeles, 1879–1939.* Berkeley: University of California Press, 2006.

Montejano, David. *Anglos and Mexicans in the Making of Texas.* Austin: University of Texas Press, 1987.

Moran, Jeffrey P. "'Modernism Gone Mad': Sex Education Comes to Chicago, 1913." *Journal of American History* 83, no. 2 (1996): 481–513.

———. *Teaching Sex: The Shaping of Adolescence in the Twentieth Century.* Cambridge, MA: Harvard University Press, 2000.

Mrozek, Donald J. "From National Health to Personal Fulfillment, 1890–1940." In *Fitness in American Culture: Images of Health, Sport, and the Body, 1830–1940,* edited by Kathryn Grover, 18–46. Amherst: University of Massachusetts Press, 1989.

Mumford, Kevin J. *Interzones: Black/White Sex Districts in Chicago and New York in the Early Twentieth Century.* New York: Columbia University Press, 1997.

Myers, Gloria. *A Municipal Mother: Portland's Lola Greene Baldwin, America's First Policewoman.* Corvallis: Oregon State University Press, 1995.

Nathanson, Constance A. *Dangerous Passage: The Social Control of Sexuality in Women's Adolescence.* Philadelphia: Temple University Press, 1991.

Neuhaus, Jessamyn. "The Importance of Being Orgasmic: Sexuality, Gender, and Marital Sex Manuals in the United States, 1920–1963." *Journal of the History of Sexuality* 9, no. 4 (2000): 447–73.

Nielsen, Kim E. *Un-American Womanhood: Antiradicalism, Antifeminism, and the First Red Scare.* Columbus: Ohio State University Press, 2001.

Odem, Mary E. *Delinquent Daughters: Protecting and Policing Adolescent Female Sexuality in the United States, 1885–1920.* Chapel Hill: University of North Carolina Press, 1995.

Parker, Alison M. *Articulating Rights: Nineteenth-Century American Women on Race, Reform, and the State.* DeKalb: Northern Illinois Press, 2010.

———. *Purifying America: Women, Cultural Reform, and Pro-censorship Activism, 1873–1933.* Urbana: University of Illinois Press, 1997.

Pascoe, Peggy. *Relations of Rescue: The Search for Female Moral Authority in the American West, 1874–1939.* New York: Oxford University Press, 1990.

Peiss, Kathy. *Cheap Amusements: Working Women and Leisure in Turn-of-the-Century New York.* Philadelphia: Temple University Press, 1986.

Pernick, Martin. *The Black Stork: Eugenics and the Death of "Defective" Babies in American Medicine and Motion Pictures since 1915.* New York: Oxford University Press, 1996.

Peterson, Paul E. *The Politics of School Reform, 1870–1940.* Chicago: University of Chicago Press, 1985.

Pickens, Donald. *Eugenics and the Progressives.* Nashville, TN: Vanderbilt Press, 1968.

Pierce, Jennifer Burek. *What Adolescents Ought to Know: Sexual Health Texts in Early Twentieth-Century America.* Amherst: University of Massachusetts Press, 2011.

Piper, John F. *The American Churches in World War I.* Athens: Ohio University Press, 1985.

Pivar, David. *Purity and Hygiene: Women, Prostitution, and the "American Plan," 1900–1930.* Westport, CT: Greenwood Press, 2002.

———. *Purity Crusade: Sexuality, Morality, and Social Control, 1868–1900.* Westport, CT: Greenwood Press, 1973.

Porter, Roy, and Lesley Hall. *The Facts of Life: The Creation of Sexual Knowledge in Britain.* New Haven, CT: Yale University Press, 1995.

Reilly, Philip. *The Surgical Solution: A History of Involuntary Sterilization in the United States.* Baltimore: Johns Hopkins University Press, 1991.

Roberts, Dorothy E. *Killing the Black Body: Race, Reproduction, and the Meaning of Liberty.* New York: Pantheon Books, 1997.

Robertson, Nancy Marie. *Christian Sisterhood, Race Relations, and the YWCA, 1906–1946.* Champaign: University of Illinois Press, 2007.

Robinson, Charles F., II. *Dangerous Liaisons: Sex and Love in the Segregated South.* Fayetteville: University of Arkansas Press, 2003.

Rodrique, Jessie M. "The Black Community and the Birth Control Movement." In *Passion and Power: Sexuality in History,* edited by Christina Simmons, 138–54. Philadelphia: Temple University Press, 1989.

Roediger, David. *The Wages of Whiteness: Race and the Making of the American Working Class.* London: Verso, 1991.

Rooks, Noliwe M. *Ladies' Pages: African American Women's Magazines and the Culture That Made Them.* New Brunswick, NJ: Rutgers University Press, 2004.

Rosenberg, Charles, and Janet Golden, eds. *Framing Disease: Studies in Cultural History.* New Brunswick, NJ: Rutgers University Press, 1992.

Rossiter, Margaret W. *Women Scientists in America.* Vol. 1, *Struggles and Strategies to 1940.* Baltimore: Johns Hopkins University Press, 1982.

Rotskoff, Lori. "Sex in the Schools: Adolescence, Sex Education, and Social Reform." *Reviews in American History* 29, no. 2 (2001): 310–18.

Rotundo, E. Anthony. *American Manhood: Transformations in Masculinity from the Revolution to the Modern Era.* New York: Basic Books, 1993.

Rupp, Leila J. *A Desired Past: A Short History of Same-Sex Love in America.* Chicago: University of Chicago Press, 2002.

San Miguel, Guadalupe. *Let All of Them Take Heed: Mexican Americans and the Campaign for Educational Equality in Texas, 1910–1981.* Austin: University of Texas Press, 1987.

Sappol, Michael. "'Morbid Curiosity': The Decline and Fall of the Popular Anatomical Museum." *Common-Place* 4, no. 2 (2004), http://www.common-place.org/vol-04/no-02/sappol/.

Schechter, Patricia Ann. *Ida B. Wells-Barnett and American Reform, 1880–1930.* Chapel Hill: University of North Carolina Press, 2001.

Schoen, Johanna. *Choice and Coercion: Birth Control, Sterilization, and Abortion in Public Health and Welfare.* Chapel Hill: University of North Carolina Press, 2005.

Sethna, Christabelle. "The Facts of Life: The Sex Instruction of Ontario Public School Children, 1900–1950." PhD diss., University of Toronto, 1995.

Shah, Nayan. *Contagious Divides: Epidemics and Race in San Francisco's Chinatown.* Berkeley: University of California Press, 2001.

Shaw, Stephanie. *What a Woman Ought to Be and to Do: Black Professional Women Workers during the Jim Crow Era.* Chicago: University of Chicago Press, 1996.

Shenk, Gerald E. *Work or Fight! Race, Gender and the Draft in World War I.* New York: Palgrave, 2005.

Simmons, Christina. "African Americans and Sexual Victorianism in the Social Hygiene Movement, 1910–1940." *Journal of the History of Sexuality* 4, no. 1 (1993): 51–75.

———. "'Modern Marriage' for African Americans, 1920–1940." *Canadian Review of American Studies* 30, no. 3 (2000): 273–300.

Skloot, Rebecca. *The Immortal Life of Henrietta Lacks.* New York: Crown, 2010.

Skocpol, Theda. *Protecting Soldiers and Mothers: The Political Origins of Social Policy in the United States.* Cambridge, MA: Belknap Press, 1992.

Smith, Susan L. *Sick and Tired of Being Sick and Tired: Black Women's Health Activism in America, 1890–1950.* Philadelphia: University of Pennsylvania Press, 1995.

Smith-Rosenberg, Carroll. *Disorderly Conduct: Visions of Gender in Victorian America.* New York: Alfred A. Knopf, 1985.

Smith-Rosenberg, Carroll, and Charles Rosenberg. "The Female Animal: Medical and Biological Views of Woman and Her Role in Nineteenth-Century America." *Journal of American History* 60, no. 2 (1973): 332–56.

Spector, Ronald H. "Josephus Daniels, Franklin Roosevelt, and the Reinvention of the Naval Enlisted Man." In *FDR and the U.S. Navy*, edited by Edward J. Marolda, 19–33. New York: St. Martin's Press, 1998.

Spring, Joel. *The American School 1642–1990*. 2nd ed. New York: Longman, 1990.

Spurlock, John C. *Free Love: Marriage and Middle-Class Radicalism in America, 1825–1860*. New York: New York University Press, 1988.

Stansell, Christine. *American Moderns: Bohemian New York and the Creation of a New Century*. New York: Metropolitan Books, 2000.

Stepan, Nancy. *The Idea of Race in Science: Great Britain 1800–1960*. London: Macmillan Press, 1982.

Stern, Alexandra Minna. *Eugenic Nation: Faults and Frontiers of Better Breeding in Modern America*. Berkeley: University of California Press, 2005.

Stewart, Ruth Ann. *Portia: The Life of Portia Washington Pittman, the Daughter of Booker T. Washington*. Garden City, NY: Doubleday, 1977.

Stoler, Laura Ann. *Race and the Education of Desire*. Durham, NC: Duke University Press, 1995.

Sullivan, Michael Anne. "Healing Bodies and Saving the Race: Women, Public Health, Eugenics, and Sexuality, 1890–1950." PhD diss., University of New Mexico, 2001.

Thomas, Robert David. *The Man Who Would Be Perfect: John Humphrey Noyes and the Utopian Impulse*. Philadelphia: University of Pennsylvania Press, 1977.

"The Two Paths." (Illustration from *Social Purity, or, the Life of the Home and Nation*, 1903). Library of Congress. American Women: The General Collections. HQ31.G46. Accessed April 15, 2006. http://memory.loc.gov/ammem/awhhtml/awgc1/d18.html.

Tyack, David, and Larry Cuban. *Tinkering toward Utopia: A Century of Public School Reform*. Cambridge, MA: Harvard University Press, 1995.

Ullman, Sharon R. *Sex Seen: The Emergence of Modern Sexuality in America*. Berkeley: University of California Press, 1997.

United States House of Representatives Committee on Government Reform—Minority Staff. *The Content of Federally Funded Abstinence-Only Education Programs* (Report Prepared for Rep. Henry A. Waxman). 2004.

Vandiver, Frank E. *Black Jack: The Life and Times of John J. Pershing*. 2 vols. College Station: Texas A&M Press, 1977.

Vaughan, Megan. *Curing Their Ills: Colonial Power and African Illness*. Stanford: Stanford University Press, 1991.

Verbrugge, Martha H. *Active Bodies: A History of Women's Physical Education in Twentieth-Century America*. New York: Oxford University Press, 2012.

Walkowitz, Judith. *Prostitution and Victorian Society: Women, Class, and the State*. Cambridge: Cambridge University Press, 1980.

Walsh, Frank. *Sin and Censorship: The Catholic Church and the Motion Picture Industry*. New Haven, CT: Yale University Press, 1996.

Walters, Pamela Barnhouse, and Philip J. O'Connell. "The Family Economy, Work, and Educational Participation in the United States, 1890–1940." *American Journal of Sociology* 93, no. 5 (1988): 116–52.

Walters, Ronald G. *Primers for Prudery: Sexual Advice to Victorian America*. Englewood Cliffs, NJ: Prentice-Hall, 1973.

Washington, Harriet A. *Medical Apartheid: The Dark History of Medical Experimentation on Black Americans from Colonial Times to the Present.* New York: Doubleday, 2006.

Welter, Barbara. "The Cult of True Womanhood, 1820–1860." *American Quarterly* 18, no. 2 (1966): 151–74.

Wheeler, Leigh Ann. "Rescuing Sex from Prudery and Prurience: American Women's Use of Sex Education as an Antidote to Obscenity, 1925–1932." *Journal of Women's History* 12, no. 3 (2000): 173–95.

White, Deborah Gray. *Too Heavy a Load: Black Women in Defense of Themselves, 1894–1994.* New York: W. W. Norton, 1999.

White, Kevin. *The First Sexual Revolution: The Emergence of Male Heterosexuality in Modern America.* New York: New York University Press, 1993.

Wiebe, Robert. *The Search for Order, 1877–1920.* New York: Hill and Wang, 1967.

Wiley, Bell Irvin. *The Life of Billy Yank: The Common Soldier of the Union.* Baton Rouge: Louisiana State University Press, 1952.

———. *The Life of Johnny Reb: The Common Soldier of the Confederacy.* Baton Rouge: Louisiana State University Press, 1943.

Woloch, Nancy. *Women and the American Experience.* New York: McGraw-Hill, 1994.

Woodward, C. Vann. *The Burden of Southern History.* Baton Rouge: Louisiana State University Press, 1960.

———. *Origins of the New South, 1877–1913.* Baton Rouge: Louisiana State University, 1951.

Woollacott, Angela. "'Khaki Fever' and Its Control: Gender, Class, Age and Sexual Morality on the British Homefront in the First World War." *Journal of Contemporary History* 29, no. 2 (1994): 325–47.

Young, Hugh. *Hugh Young: A Surgeon's Autobiography.* New York: Harcourt, Brace, 1940.

Young, James Harvey. *The Toadstool Millionaires: A Social History of Patent Medicines in America before Federal Regulation.* Princeton, NJ: Princeton University Press, 1961.

Zeitz, Joshua. *Flapper: A Madcap Story of Sex, Style, Celebrity, and the Women Who Made America Modern.* New York: Three Rivers Press, 2006.

Zimmerman, Jonathan. *Distilling Democracy: Alcohol Education in America's Public Schools, 1880–1925.* Lawrence: University Press of Kansas, 1999.

Index